Ophthalmic Electrodiagnosis

Volume 1 in the Series

Major Problems in Ophthalmology

PATRICK D. TREVOR-ROPER, FRCS
Consulting Editor

OTHER MONOGRAPHS IN THE SERIES

PUBLISHED

Watson and Hazleman: **The Sclera & Systemic Disorders**

FORTHCOMING

Easty, Carter and Richmond: **Virus Disease of the Eye**

Ophthalmic Electrodiagnosis

N. R. GALLOWAY, MD, FRCS

Consultant Ophthalmologist, and
Clinical Teacher in Ophthalmology, Nottingham University
Medical School.

Second edition

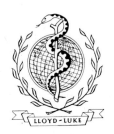

LLOYD-LUKE (Medical Books) LTD.
49 NEWMAN STREET · LONDON

1981

OPTOMETRY

FILMSET, PRINTED AND BOUND IN GREAT BRITAIN BY
HAZELL WATSON AND VINEY LTD
AYLESBURY, BUCKS

ISBN 0 85324 152 X

Foreword

The primary aim of our monographs on Major Problems in Ophthalmology is to cover those aspects of the speciality where there have been many recent advances, with which the larger book cannot hope to keep pace. Those subjects which are readily omitted in the standard text-books, either because they overlap into neighbouring medical disciplines, or else because they require special background knowledge, to which a hurried chapter in a standard compendium can do scant justice, also fall within our brief.

This, the first of our series on Ophthalmic Electrodiagnosis, falls happily into both these categories. Among our many recent acquisitions in ophthalmology has been a proper understanding of the complex electrical changes in the retina and optic pathways, together with their potential value in assessing retinal function, especially in eyes where the view of the retina is obscured or where the evident damage is difficult to interpret. At the same time techniques have been refined and tests elaborated which greatly enhance our diagnostic capacity in this respect.

Nicholas Galloway offers us a comprehensive and cogent account of his subject, leading us patiently through the complex issues, and culminating in valuable advice on the setting-up of such a unit in small or large departments. Those of us whose understanding of electrophysics is apt to be shaky will be especially grateful for so readable and helpful a guide.

London, 1975   PATRICK TREVOR-ROPER

Preface to Second Edition

Since the first edition was published there have been several advances in the field of ocular electrodiagnosis especially in relation to the Visually Evoked Potential. The chapter on this subject has been expanded to include some of the more recent work relating the VEP to changes in the visual field and visual acuity. Like the first edition, the second edition is intended to be a basic guide for all those working in the field of ocular electrodiagnosis. The emphasis is on the side of clinical Ophthalmology and it is hoped that non-clinicians as well as postraduate ophthalmologists during their training will find it helpful. Much of the original form of the book has been maintained although more up-to-date references have been added throughout and several new illustrations have been included.

Nottingham
October, 1980

N. R. GALLOWAY

Preface to First Edition

The aim of this book is to show that electrodiagnosis as applied to the eye is no longer a subject which is limited to the laboratory, nor should its application be confined to a few specialised centres. It is only by widespread use and familiarity that the full clinical potential of the methods will be developed.

Better communication between the two disciplines, physics and clinical medicine, has led to the appearance of electronic equipment both in the wards and in the outpatient clinics. The application of electrodiagnostic techniques to ophthalmology has undergone an expansion, and many people would be surprised at the number of papers published every year on the subject. This provides the first problem when writing a book of this sort; it is likely to be out of date by the time it is published. There is another problem; that of presenting a speciality in a form palatable to the non-specialists. I have attempted to deal with both these problems, but I am aware that much new data will be available by the time this book goes to press. Much of the material may seem naive to the specialist and at the same time too technical to the non-specialist. The book is directed at the postgraduate student but also at the ophthalmologist or physicist who is concerned with organising an electro-diagnostic clinic of this type.

It seemed logical to divide the book into two parts and the reader will see that the first part concerns the theoretical background of these electrodiagnostic tests, whereas the second part is concerned with their clinical application. In the past a large part of the work of electrodiagnostic clinics has been concerned with the investigation of pigmentary retinopathies. For this reason it will be seen that the chapter on Inherited Retinal Disease is rather longer than the others. It seemed better to preserve this subject as a whole rather than attempt to maintain a more even balance of chapters. On the other hand, the chapter on the Visually Evoked Response must be considered rather short if this relatively new technique is to be seen in its true perspective. This is entirely due to my own limited experience in this field.

ACKNOWLEDGEMENTS

Much of the information in this book has been gained from the experience of running an electrodiagnostic clinic and this was in turn made possible by the financial help of the Sheffield Regional Hospital Board, now known as the Trent Area Health Authority. I am most grateful for this. I would also like to thank all those people who have given individual assistance and advice. In particular I am more than grateful to Mrs H. Ashcroft for her indefatigable help with typing and references, and to Mrs Lewis, the librarian of the Nottingham General Hospital for her efficient library service. The illustrations have been almost without exception drawn and prepared by Mr Lyth, the medical artist at the General Hospital. My thanks are also due to Professor A. T. Birmingham for his painstaking reading of the manuscript and for his helpful advice. Mr Colin Barber has given invaluable help on the chapters dealing more closely with medical physics and the writing of this part of the book would have been impossible without his wide technical knowledge. I would like to thank my colleagues at the Eye Hospital for sending me interesting cases, some of which are mentioned in this book. I am indebted to Dr G. B. Arden and Dr J. Kelsey for originally cultivating my interest in electrodiagnostics at the electrodiagnostic clinic in Moorfields Eye Hospital, London and for numerous helpful discussions in past years. Finally I would like to thank Mr Inglis of W. B. Saunders Company Ltd for his advice and help with the proofs and Mr P. D. Trevor-Roper for inviting me to contribute to his series of monographs. It would not be possible to end without acknowledging the forbearance of my family who have shown so much patience and equanimity.

Nottingham, 1975   N. R. GALLOWAY

Contents

PART ONE

The Method and Theory of Electrodiagnostic Techniques as Applied to the Eye

CHAPTER ONE

Basic Electronics

A detailed knowledge of electronics is not an essential background for the understanding of clinical electrodiagnostic tests any more than an accurate knowledge of the workings of a motor car engine is necessary in order to be able to drive a car. On the other hand, if the clinician is to become fully conversant with the possible sources of error in his equipment, then a working knowledge of electronics is essential. In this book it is assumed that the reader has the basic knowledge of physics required for the average medical school. Those who feel well versed in this subject should skip this chapter since it is intended only as a brief and elementary refresher course about the nature of electricity. An explanation of some unfamiliar terms or concepts may be found in the glossary at the end of this chapter. Several textbooks on electronics for medical purposes have been published, e.g. Tammes, A. R. (1971) *Electronics for Medical and Biology Laboratory Personnel*, Baltimore, Maryland: Williams and Wilkins Co.; Strong, P. (1970) *Biophysical Measurements*, Beaverton, Oregon: Tektronix Inc.

THE NATURE OF ELECTRICITY

An electric current is simply the movement of electric charge from one place to another. Some materials, such as metals, allow this to occur easily; others, such as plastic, resist the flow of electric current. Good conductors of electricity are made up of atoms which have 'loose' electrons in their outer orbits which can easily be displaced. Consecutive displacement of loose electrons in a conductor produces a wave of disturbance which travels at a speed approaching the speed of light. This process is termed electronic flow. In some materials, physiological materials for example, the positive ions are also free to move and the current includes a flow of electrons in one direction together with a flow of positive ions in the opposite direction. This movement of ions is termed ionic flow and one of the problems of measuring electrophysiological signals is the changeover from ionic flow to electron flow at the body/electrode interface. (Such a current will only flow if sufficient 'electrical pressure' is available and if the circuit is completed by a suitable conductor.)

Current and Voltage

Potential difference is the term used for 'electrical pressure' and the unit used is the volt. Different types of conductor offer a different amount of hindrance to the flow of electrical current and this hindrance to flow is termed resistance and measured in ohms. The flow of current is measured in amperes. It should be apparent that with a constant head of pressure, the size of the current will depend on the amount of resistance. The relationship between potential difference, current and resistance was discovered by the German scientist George Ohm. Ohm's law states that:

$$I = V/R \text{ where } I = \text{current in amperes}$$
$$V = \text{potential difference in volts}$$
$$R = \text{resistance in ohms.}$$

Direct Current and Alternating Current

When current flows at a constant rate and direction in a conductor it is termed direct current (DC). An example is the circuit of a simple electric torch when it is illuminated. Nowadays many power sources produce a constantly varying current; the domestic electricity supply in the UK for example has a current which flows to and fro at 50 cycles per second. This is known as alternating current (AC). Alternating current differs in certain other ways from direct current. The hindrance to flow in this case is not limited to resistance but includes other factors which limit the breaking down and building up of current and are known as inductance and capacitance. The total limiting effect of resistance, inductance and capacitance is called the impedance. In biological electronics we are nearly always dealing with alternating current although this may be sometimes superimposed on a direct current. Ohm's law can be extended to AC circuits provided all the factors hindering the flow of current are taken into account. We then have:

$$I = V/Z \text{ where } Z = \text{impedance in ohms.}$$

Bioelectric Potential

This may be defined as the electrical pressure difference between the inside and the outside of a cell. This is the potential difference across the cell wall. All cells show this resting potential, which may amount to about 90 mV. In some cells a marked change in this potential may occur when the cell is stimulated and this may cause an electric current to flow in the surrounding region. At this point one must distinguish between the kind of electric current which flows in electrical apparatus and that which flows in living tissue. Bioelectric currents are due to the movement of positive and negative ions rather than electrons, and as these ions possess finite mass and encounter resistance to movement within a conducting fluid, their speeds are limited compared with the flow of electric current in a wire. Because bioelectric potentials are often small—in the region of one mV or less—they must be magnified by means of an amplifier before they can be detected by a suitable recording instrument such as a penwriter or an oscilloscope. The small size of the recorded potential is partly due to the fact that it may have to be picked up from a site remote from its source.

Electrical Noise

Noise is the name given to any form of interference which distorts the true form of the recorded bioelectric potential change. Three important types of noise are encountered. Perhaps the most important is mains hum which is due to mains frequency interference and its harmonics. The human body can act as a radio aerial and pick up mains hum from the mains wiring in the walls of the house or hospital. Therefore, when several wires are connected to the body in order to detect potential changes, mains hum can be picked up in all of them and is thus common to them all. Interference which is common to all leads is termed the 'common mode signal'. Another form of noise is random noise, comparable with the hiss heard from a record player when the volume is turned up. Random noise arises from the electronic circuitry of the equipment. Finally, extraneous biological noise must be distinguished from the particular signal that is being investigated. There are several ways of eliminating noise; these include screening, filtering, the use of differential amplifiers and averaging. Screening and filtering can be useful for eliminating mains hum and other external sources of interference by preventing them from reaching the equipment. It is important to realise that filtering must be used with care or part of the signal may also be removed. In practice the usefulness of filters is generally limited to removing high-frequency random noise. The differential amplifier is specifically designed to reduce the strength of the common mode signal. Averaging devices are designed to detect a wanted signal amongst extraneous biological noise.

GLOSSARY

Active electrode. One of two inputs other than the earth connection of a differential amplifier. This is applied as closely as possible to the source of the potential being investigated.

Ampere. A unit of current. For biological measurements the normal flow is measured in microamperes (μA).

Amplifier. An electronic device for enlarging the size of a signal.

Bandwidth. Signals of many different frequencies are represented in the action potential of a cell or group of cells. In practice all or most of the electroretinogram signal is represented within a bandwidth from zero to 10 000 Hz. Reducing the bandwidth accepted by the amplifier reduces the noise in the signal.

Biphasic response. A twin response with components of opposite polarity.

Bipolar recording. The name given to the arrangement of the terminals of a differential amplifier.

Common mode rejection ratio. A measure of the ability of a differential amplifier to amplify the required signal and reject the common mode signal. Thus:

$$Common\ mode\ rejection\ ratio\ =\ \frac{\text{gain of amplifier for differential signal}}{\text{gain of amplifier for common mode signal}}$$

For a good amplifier the common mode rejection ratio might be 100 000:1. The 'common mode rejection' is the ratio expressed in decibels. Thus, if the common mode rejection ratio is 100 000:1 then the common mode rejection = 20×log of ratio = 100 dB (decibels).

Current limiting. Under normal conditions the current flowing through the electrodes of a biological amplifier is very small. If the amplifier were faulty, this current could increase to dangerous levels; current limiting implies the incorporation of a device to prevent any such increase.

Depolarisation. A term referring to the electrical changes which occur in a cell after it has been stimulated.

Differential amplifier. An amplifier with two inputs which amplifies the signal across those inputs and rejects any signal present in both (e.g. mains interference).

Earth. The zero level to which all potentials are referred. In most electronic equipment the terminals of any components which are to be kept at this level are connected to the chassis of the instrument and this in turn is connected to a metal conductor in contact with the ground, such as a water pipe.

Electrode. The means of making electrical contact with the body. The choice of electrode material is important in electrodiagnostic procedures since an unsuitable type of electrode can behave like a small battery when in contact with the skin. This may result in the addition of a small but unpredictable DC component to the signal.

Electrode jelly. Saline-based jelly used to ensure good contact between electrodes and skin.

Frequency. The number of waves per second, measured in cycles/second or Hertz (Hz).

Hum. A type of noise in particular mains frequency interference and its harmonics.

Impedance. The equivalent of resistance in an AC circuit.

Indifferent electrode. The other input to a differential amplifier (see 'active electrode'). The signal between active and indifferent electrode is measured.

Lead. Any wire entering or leaving a component.

Load. The impedance of the circuit into which a signal is being fed.

Microprocessor. The 'computer on a chip'. A central processing unit (CPU), of minicomputer power, produced as a single integrated circuit. Other chips are needed for programme memory and data memory to form a working system, usually on a single circuit board. The term microprocessor may refer just to the CPU or to the whole board.

Open circuit. Usually refers to a defect in the leads or components producing a break in electrical continuity.

Phase difference. The temporal relationship between different waves or different points on the same curve. It is usually expressed as an angular measure in fractions of a cycle (one cycle = 360° or 2π radians).

Photoelectric cell. A device that shows a change in its resistance when light or other electromagnetic radiations strike it. In electroretinography it is usual for the stimulus to be recorded simultaneously through a photocell and the resulting electrical impulse is used as a stimulus marker.

Power supply. The circuit that provides various levels of voltage and current for other circuits or electronic devices.

Rectify. To convert AC to DC.

Signal. An information-bearing electrical change.

Stimulus artefact. An extraneous electrical change picked up by the recording electrodes and produced by the stimulus equipment.

Transformer. A device consisting of two unconnected coils or windings which when current flows in one coil, will induce a voltage in the second coil.

X–Y recorder. A device used to plot two variables against one another on chart paper. It is a useful additional instrument in the electrodiagnostic clinic where extreme accuracy is required.

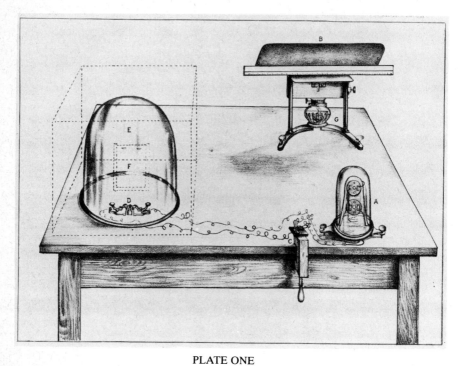

PLATE ONE

Electroretinography in the eighteen seventies (from Dewar & McKendrick, 1873).

CHAPTER TWO

The Electroretinogram

The study of electrical changes in the eye has now been in progress for more than a hundred years, and electrophysiological measurements on the eye are now becoming part of our clinical routine. In the early years these studies were largely confined to experimental animals, but there is now an international society of clinical electroretinography which has been in existence for over 20 years. The first work in this field was concerned with the corneo-retinal potential, or the resting potential. This may be defined as the difference in potential between the cornea and the posterior pole of the eye. It was first described by Emil DuBois Reymond, professor of physiology in Berlin (DuBois Reymond, 1849). He showed that the cornea is electrically positive with respect to the posterior pole; however, it was not until 16 years later that Holmgren observed that the resting potential can be modified by the action of light shining on the retina (Holmgren, 1865). Shortly after this, Dewar and McKendrick, working in Edinburgh, rediscovered this light response quite independently and they only came upon Holmgren's paper after their own results had been published (Dewar and McKendrick, 1873). They were able to show that the changes in potential on impact of light amounted to three to ten per cent of the normal resting potential and were independent of the anterior portion of the eye. Initially their experiments were carried out by placing electrodes on the cornea and the posterior pole of the eye, but they subsequently showed that the response to light could also be recorded between the exposed brain and the cornea allowing the eye to be left *in situ*. They then found that the same electrical changes could be recorded by placing electrodes on the cornea and an adjacent area of skin. Having made this discovery they were able to attempt to produce a human electroretinogram; this was achieved by using a clay trough filled with saline as the corneal electrode. These early attempts at human electroretinography were far from satisfactory and Dewar and McKendrick concluded that "the method is too exhausting and uncertain to permit of qualitative observations being made".

THE EVOLUTION OF ELECTRORETINOGRAPHY

At the turn of the century considerable advances were made in the techniques of recording electrical responses in animals. In 1903 Gotch, working in the physiological laboratory at Oxford, recorded responses from excised frogs' eyes, measuring them with a capillary electrometer and using an arc lamp as stimulus. He was able to photograph his records and he found that the positive component of the electroretinogram measured up to 0·001 V and was preceded by a slight dip of negativity (Gotch, 1903). It was known therefore at the turn of the century that a biphasic type of response could be produced by a single flash of light. At the same time it was being shown that a similar response could be demonstrated in a wide range of vertebrates. In 1908 Einthoven and Jolly showed the presence of a third and later component in the electroretinogram, the positive 'c' wave. The negative and positive waves preceding this have been known as the 'a' and 'b' waves respectively (Einthoven and Jolly, 1908) (Figure 2.1).

The introduction of the valve amplifier brought about a dramatic improvement in recording techniques and led to a further understanding of the origin and nature of the response. In 1925 Hartline carried out a series of detailed experiments confirming that the response from intact animals was identical to that obtained from excised open eyes (Hartline, 1925). Four years later, Sachs was able to show that the human electroretinogram was typically dependent on the scotopic visual system of the retina and that the electroretinogram of protanopes was relatively reduced in red light. At this point we had reached the stage when a waveform could be accurately recorded and measured, and it was known beyond doubt that this waveform was produced by the retina, even though it was recorded through electrodes which were placed at some distance from the eye. In the early 1930s, attempts were being made to record the human electroretinogram using the valve amplifier, but at the same time

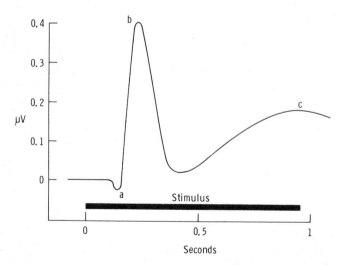

Figure 2.1. Diagram to illustrate a vertebrate electroretinogram obtained using a pen recorder. Note the three waves and their time and amplitude relationships.

an important milestone was reached in the study of responses from animals. This was the classical work of Granit on cats. He developed the ideas put forward by Einthoven and Jolly after the turn of the century, suggesting that the electroretinogram represents the sum of three waveforms which he termed 'processes'. These he enumerated as PI, PII, and PIII. He showed that if the electroretinogram is recorded from a cat subjected to deepening levels of ether anaesthesia, the waveform changes in a characteristic manner. This change in waveform was thought to be due to the selective inhibition of each of the three processes, PI, PII and PIII, in turn. Although they have been elaborated to some extent, these original ideas about the nature of the electroretinogram are still held to be true today (Granit, 1933).

As soon as the knowledge of the basic components had become well established, much interest was centred on the relative contribution of photopic and scotopic mechanisms to the response. In 1940 Bernhard noted that the flicker fusion frequency was not the same under photopic and scotopic conditions. This difference is now used in many electrodiagnostic clinics to assess cone function (Bernhard, 1940). In 1946 Adrian showed that the electroretinogram can be split into fast and slow components, the former present in the light-adapted eye and more prominent in red light, and the latter more prominent after dark adaptation and using light of a shorter wavelength. Under suitable conditions the two responses were superimposed, producing double-humped 'a' and 'b' waves.

THE CONTACT LENS ELECTRODE

Although it can be seen that considerable advances in our understanding of the electrical responses from the eye were made from work on animals, investigations on human subjects had always been hampered by the technical problem of fixing the electrodes. A great step forward was made in 1941 when Riggs introduced the contact lens electrode. Until this time clinical electroretinography did not really exist and little was known about alterations in disease. In fact the use of the contact lens remained in abeyance during the war years until the pioneering work of Karpe began to be published from Stockholm in 1945. It soon became apparent that the contact lens electrode eliminated much of the interference due to background noise (Riggs, 1941; Karpe, 1945).

MORE RECENTLY DISCOVERED COMPONENTS OF THE ELECTRORETINOGRAM

Using the method described by Karpe, the human electroretinogram could be recorded as a biphasic response, a negative 'a' wave was not usually seen, due to the brief duration of the stimulus. But it had been previously shown in other animals that a series of small wavelets could be sometimes seen on the 'b' wave (Frohlich, 1914; Granit, 1947). In 1954 Cobb and Morton described the phenomenon in man and named it the Oscillatory Potential. They counted four to six wavelets using a brief flash stimulus lasting 250 μsec (Cobb and Morton, 1954). Since then it has been shown that these wavelets may be selectively abolished by disease. The significance of this will be discussed in the various chapters concerned with the abnormal response.

The most recent component of importance to be discovered is the Early Receptor Potential. This is a very rapid component which can be seen at the very beginning of the response, immediately before the 'a' wave. Brown and Murakami first described it in 1964, and showed that it could only be elicited by an intense light stimulus. The latent period is very short, less than 60 μsec, and it appears as a small positive peak followed by a larger negative one. Its importance lies in the fact that it is thought to be an electrical manifestation of the bleaching of photopigment in the retina (Brown and Murakami, 1964).

ADVANCES IN RECORDING TECHNIQUE

Until recently the routine method of recording the electroretinogram entailed enlarging or amplifying the minute electrical changes picked up from corneal and skin electrodes and reproducing them on paper by some form of pen-writer. This technique was similar to routine electrocardiography. However, the use of the oscilloscope as a recording instrument now gives a more accurate response and the result can be photographed with Polaroid film. A further advance has been the introduction of the technique of averaging. Signal averaging is a valuable way of separating the true response from background interference and sometimes a response can be seen which was quite obscured in the original trace. The method involves recording a series of consecutive responses from which an average trace is obtained. The crudest way of doing this is simply to superimpose these repeated responses using a pen recorder, but a more sophisticated and more useful method entails feeding the records into a computer programmed specifically for this purpose.

THE NORMAL ELECTRORETINOGRAM

From this brief historical survey it should be apparent that our knowledge of the electrical response from the eye due to a flash of light has evolved from the time when a simple biphasic response was observed to the present more complex waveform. Not surprisingly the electroretinogram can vary considerably, depending on the type of stimulus that is used. There are also a number of other factors which influence the normal response and these are considered in more detail in Chapter 7. Using the method of recording human electroretinograms described by Karpe, the normal value of the amplitude of the 'b' waves should be about 0·3 mV (Karpe, Rickenbach and Thomasson, 1950), but it should be stressed that even with well-standardised techniques there are still wide variations in the normal values, and for clinical purposes more attention should be paid to the shape of the waveform rather than to the size of the 'b' wave in mV. It is also important to realise at this point that the shape of the waveform depends greatly on the type of stimulus used. Thus in Figure 2.2 the response to an intense stimulus is shown, but using the weaker stimulus of Karpe a different type of trace is seen (Figure 2.3). As a general rule, if the intensity is increased, then at first both the 'a' and 'b' waves increase in amplitude, but above a certain level the 'b' wave becomes saturated and does not show any further increase with increasing intensity. On the other

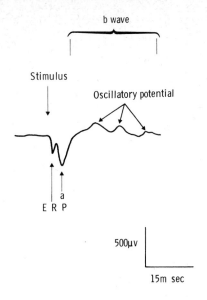

Figure 2.2. The normal response in a light-adapted eye.

hand, the 'a' wave continues to expand and thus in high intensity responses a large 'a' wave and relatively small 'b' wave are seen. Other features also appear at high intensities: the oscillatory wavelets become more evident and the Early Receptor Potential may be seen preceding the 'a' wave.

THE ORIGIN OF THE ELECTRORETINOGRAM

If the clinical value of the electroretinogram is to be fully realised in the future, a full understanding of the mode of production of the waveform will be essential. A superficial inspection of the problem might lead us to search for an origin of the 'a' wave in one layer of the retina, the 'b' wave in another, and so on. However, the wealth of research which has been carried out so far indicates that the source of the response that we record must be looked for in two stages. First we must find out what component waves are added together to produce the final response, and then secondly, having isolated these components, their anatomical site of origin must be determined. A further question arises when we consider that the electroretinogram is a mass response; is it the sum of different kinds of response from different parts of the retinal sphere? Local responses from different parts of the retina can now be obtained, at least in the laboratory (Brindley, 1956), and it is perhaps surprising that the response from a very small area of retina is very similar to the

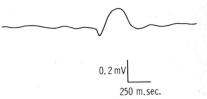

Figure 2.3. Diagram to show a typical human electroretinogram as traditionally recorded using a contact lens electrode and pen recorder. The 'c' wave, oscillatory potential and early receptor potential do not appear on this type of trace.

mass response. Differences can be seen in the waveform of records from the fovea and the peripheral retina in the Cynomolgus monkey, although they have not yet been confirmed in man. At the fovea the 'b' wave is small whereas the 'a' wave is large (Brown, 1969). It will be shown that these differences may be partly due to the fact that the rods and cones do not produce exactly the same kind of response and partly because of the different anatomical configuration of the nerve elements at the fovea and the peripheral retina.

Analysis of the Response

As long ago as the 1930s it was known that there are characteristic differences between the electroretinogram produced by a rod-dominated retina and that produced by a cone-dominated one. Figure 2.4 shows the type of response that can be obtained from the eye of a cat (rod dominated), compared with that from a light-adapted frog's eye (cone dominated). One important difference is the off-response which takes the form of a simple negative deflection in the cat electroretinogram, but appears as a positive deflection sometimes known as the 'd' wave in the light-adapted frog. It can also be seen that the 'c' wave is not present in the response from the cone-dominated retina. When Granit put forward his classical analysis of the electroretinogram he showed how three different waves, which he named PI, PII and PIII, could sum

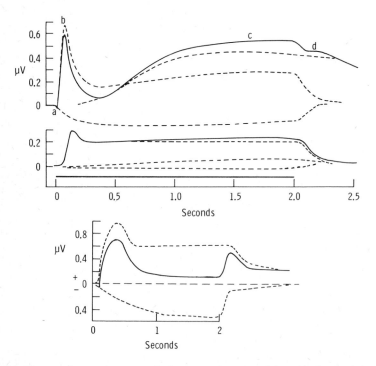

Figure 2.4. The upper trace shows a typical response from a rod-dominated retina when dark adapted. The middle trace also shows the response from a rod-dominated retina, but this time when adapted to light. The lower trace was from a cone-dominated retina. Reproduced from Granit, R. (1933) *Journal of Physiology*, **77**, 221, with permission.

together to produce an electroretinogram in the case of both rod and cone types of retina. Figure 2.5 is a diagram to illustrate this.

Evidence is now beginning to accumulate which confirms the independent nature of PI, PII and PIII, and furthermore we are beginning to learn something about their site of origin. Some of this evidence will now be considered taking each 'process' in turn.

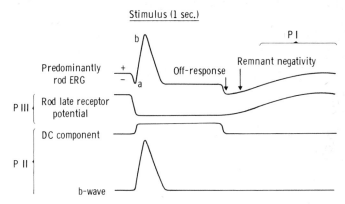

Figure 2.5. Diagram to show how Granit's three 'processes', PI, PII and PIII, summate to produce a normal electroretinogram.

PI. Granit showed that the 'c' wave of the electroretinogram behaves quite independently from the 'a' and 'b' waves and it is abolished at an early stage under ether anaesthesia in the cat (Granit, 1933). Noell showed that the 'c' wave can be selectively abolished by destroying the pigment epithelium with sodium iodate (Noell, 1954). There is other evidence which indicates that the 'c' wave cannot be recorded from the isolated retina; it therefore appears to be an independent part of the response, perhaps derived from the pigment epithelium, and the component producing it was termed 'PI' by Granit.

PII. Granit identified the positive part of the response of the 'b' wave as being due largely to this component. It is abolished at a deeper level of ether anaesthesia than PI and it also becomes selectively abolished at low stimulus intensities. More recently it has been shown that PII is composed of two parts, a positive peak represented by the 'b' wave and a more prolonged positive plateau on which the 'b' wave is superimposed. The plateau part of the response has been called the DC component. The 'b' wave and DC component behave independently under experimental conditions, but microelectrode experiments indicate that both these parts of PII arise from the inner nuclear layer (Brown and Tasaki, 1961). The development of more sophisticated microelectrode techniques has now enabled recordings to be made from a variety of individual cells in the retina. In the search for the cellular origin of the 'b' wave, Miller and Dowling found a response in the Müller cells of the mud puppy which closely resembled the 'b' wave. Although previously it had been suspected that the 'b' wave arose from the bipolars, these responses from the Müller cells (glial cells) were the only slow potentials, as opposed to spike potentials, whose latency and waveform appeared to fit the required measurements exactly (Miller and Dowling, 1970).

PIII. At deeper levels of ether anaesthesia in the cat, a negative wave is obtained. Similarly, a negative wave may be obtained in the human electro-retinogram under certain pathological conditions; for example, this may be seen after a central retinal vein occlusion. Microelectrode experiments suggest that this negative component arises from the inner segments of the receptors. The leading edge of PIII is seen as the 'a' wave in the intact electroretinogram, but the remainder of PIII is altered and obscured by superimposition of PI and PII. This component became known as the receptor potential until it was discovered that an earlier component exists prior to the 'a' wave and it is now more usual to refer to PIII as the late receptor potential. Brown and co-workers have shown how the late receptor potential is retained when the inner half of the retina is starved of its blood supply by clamping the retinal circu-lation and the 'b' wave is abolished. They have also shown that the shape of the late receptor potential is different in areas of retina where cones predomi-nate. The cone late receptor potential has a sharper cut-off compared with the rods response and Figure 2.6 illustrates how this difference can explain the different types of off-response in cone- and rod-dominated retinae respec-tively (Brown, 1969; Whitten and Brown, 1973).

ORIGIN OF THE MORE RECENTLY DISCOVERED COMPONENTS

The Oscillatory Potential

In the monkey these wavelets are abolished in a striking manner by clamping the retinal circulation (Brown, 1969), and they are also abolished in the human eye after central retinal artery occlusion. The fact that their presence appears to depend on the integrity of the retinal circulation suggests that they may arise in the inner part of the retina which receives its nourishment from this source. It is interesting, however, that the wavelets seem to be more susceptible to ischaemic change than the 'b' wave. Intraretinal microelec-trodes have been used to record oscillatory responses from the inner nuclear layer of the frog's retina and the responses can only be produced if a wide area of retina is stimulated. There is also some evidence that the wavelets are produced by tangentially orientated structures and they are particularly well seen in various vertebrates where there is a thick and well-developed inner nuclear layer (Algvere, 1968).

It has been suggested that the wavelets are related to observed cyclical changes in amplitude of the spike discharges in the optic nerve (Steinberg, 1966), and hence their origin from the ganglion cells, but they are still present in optic atrophy and antidromic stimulation of optic nerve fibres does not reset the rhythm of the wavelets. There is no doubt that the wavelets can be best produced by exposing the eye to double flashes spaced about 15 seconds apart. The second flash tends to produce a more well-defined response and this requirement for preadaptation becomes more marked when the eye is dark adapted. The maximum chromatic sensitivity of the wavelets has been shown to be at the red end of the spectrum and it has also been claimed that the wavelets are abolished in patients with congenital achromatopsia. Their exact site of origin is therefore still in doubt although the evidence at present seems to point to the inner nuclear layer. In view of the fact that the wavelets show certain features in common with a response recordable from the ama-

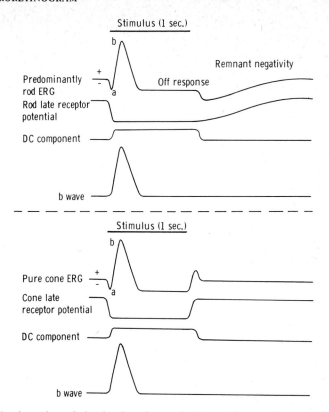

Figure 2.6. A schematic analysis of rod- and cone-dominated electroretinograms which shows how the different shapes of the rod and cone late receptor potentials (PIII) influence the final trace. Brown, K. T. (1969) In 'The Electroretinograms', from *The Retina: Morphology, Function and Clinical Characteristics* (Eds.) Straatsma, B., Hull, M., Alba, R. & Crescitelli, F., p. 352, Figure 163. Originally published by the University of California Press; reprinted by permission of The Regent of the University of California.

crine cells it has been suggested that they could represent a feedback mechanism from the amacrines to the bipolars (Algarve and Westbeck, 1972).

More recently it has been found that the last of the oscillatory potentials appears to behave in a different way to the others. Its timing alters with increase in stimulus frequency in a different manner. In fact the last wavelet appears to be time-locked to the stimulus offset, whereas the others are not. The suggestion is that the last wavelet is part of the off-response, being generated by the retinal off elements described in single cell recordings. (Kojima and Zrenner 1978; Wachtmeister and Dowling 1977).

The Early Receptor Potential

Although the latent period of the 'a' wave becomes much shorter with stronger stimuli, it is never less than about 2 msec and for some years before 1964 it was suspected that a response might exist which bridged the gap between the moment of excitation and the onset of PIII. In 1964 Brown and Murakami found that an electrical response of no detectable latency could be recorded from a microelectrode inserted into the inner segment of the receptors (Brown and Murakami, 1964). It was then shown that this rapid biphasic response could be recorded with large electrodes outside the retina and in fact it can now be recorded as a routine clinical procedure in the human. The action spectrum of this response agrees with that for bleaching visual pigment. The early receptor potential has been elusive in the past because it is easily obscured by artefacts and a strong flash is required to elicit it. However, it is now known to be biphasic; a small positive component known as R_1 is followed by a larger negative component known as R_2. R_2 leads directly into the 'a' wave. Because the latency is virtually zero, both R_1 and R_2 are thought to

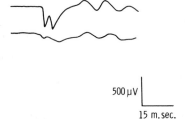

Figure 2.7. From above downwards the first and second responses at half-minute intervals to an intense stimulus. The early receptor potential and the remainder of the response are just beginning to recover again in the lower trace.

500 µV

15 m.sec.

arise from the outer segments of the receptors and it has been suggested that they are due to movements of charge in visual pigment molecules. The early receptor potential is more resistant to disease than the other components of the electroretinogram and when recorded from the isolated retina it is not much altered by formaldehyde or metal chelating agents. On heating the retina it disappears at the same temperature at which the regular orientation of the pigment molecules is lost (Brindley and Gardner Medwin, 1966; Cone and Brown, 1967).

When recording the human early receptor potential the type of stimulus flash that is used produces a dense after-image which fades and changes colour over a period of about two minutes. If the flash is immediately repeated, when the after-image is still very dense, no response is obtained, but it may be elicited again after about a quarter of a minute (see Figure 2.7). The early receptor potential is therefore photolabile and this distinguishes it from certain other electrical effects which can be produced by flashing a strong light on other tissues. For example, a change in electrical potential which is not photolabile can be recorded from the pigment epithelium after the retina has been removed.

The relative contributions to the response by rods and cones have been investigated by measuring the amplitude of the early receptor potential when evoked by different coloured lights. A maximal response is shown by using a flash with a wavelength of 530 nm but at higher intensities a more blue light is required. This could suggest that rods contribute more to the response at higher intensities. Another approach has been by measuring the recovery time of the early receptor potential. For example, after a red flash the early receptor potential recovers more rapidly than after a blue one. The recovery half-time after a red flash is in the region of 100 sec; after a blue flash the recovery half-time is in the region of 200 sec. These measurements fit in well with densitometric measurements of recovery times of rod and cone pigments (Francois et al, 1974).

RELATIONSHIP BETWEEN VISUAL EXCITATION AND THE ELECTRORETINOGRAM

A different approach to the study of the origin of the electroretinogram has entailed the recording of responses to light from the outer segments of small pieces of isolated retina using microelectrodes. Accurate positioning of the microelectrodes can be achieved under direct vision by infra-red microscopy. Using such a technique, Penn and Hagins have described a steady electric current which flows in the interstitial space of the receptor layer of the retina and enters the rod outer segments in darkness. When the rods are illuminated by a flash of light, the dark current is immediately reduced. The light-induced change has been termed the photocurrent. This current has been found to be large enough to account for the ability of the retina to respond to single photons absorbed in the rod outer segments and its behaviour resembles the 'a' wave and PIII component of the electroretinogram (Penn and Hagins, 1972).

SUMMARY

1. Although the electroretinogram can be recorded through electrodes placed outside and even at a distance from the eye, there is no doubt that it is produced by the retina, and other structures in and around the eye probably make no contribution to it.

2. The electroretinogram is made up of the following components: the early receptor potential, the 'a' wave, the 'b' wave, and the 'c' wave. There is also an 'off effect' whose position depends on the timing of the stimulus flash.

3. The early receptor potential is thought to arise from the outer segments of the receptors, the 'a' wave is part of Granit's PIII component, and this is thought to arise from the inner segments of the receptors. The 'b' wave corresponds to Granit's PII component and this is thought to arise from the inner nuclear layer and possibly from the Müller cells. The 'c' wave which corresponds with PI probably arises from the pigment epithelium. Under suitable stimulus conditions, the 'b' wave is modified by the appearance of three or four small wavelets which probably arise in the inner nuclear layer, but not from the same source as the 'b' wave itself. These wavelets are particularly sensitive to pathological changes in the retina.

REFERENCES

Adrian, E. D. (1945) The electric response of the human eye. *Journal of Physiology*, **104**, 84–104.

Algvere, P. (1968) Studies on the oscillatory potential of the clinical electroretinogram. *Acta Ophthalmologica (København)*, Suppl. **96**, 1–33.

Algvere, P. & Westbeck, S. (1972) Human electrogram in response to double flashes of light during the course of dark adaptation. *Vision Research*, **12**, 195–214.

Bernhard, C. G. (1940) Contributions to the neurophysiology of the optic pathway. *Acta Physiologica Scandinavica*, **1**, Supp. 1.

Brindley, G. S. (1956) The effect on the frog's electroretinogram of varying the amount of retina illuminated. *Journal of Physiology*, **134**, 353–359.

Brindley, G. S. & Gardner Medwin, A. R. (1966) The origin of the early receptor potential. *Journal of Physiology*, **182**, 185–194.

Brown, K. T. (1969) The electroretinogram, its components and their origins. In *The Retina: Morphology, Function and Clinical Characteristics*. pp. 319–368. (Ed.) Straatsma, B., Hull, M., Alba, R. & Crescitelli, F. California: University of California Forum for Medical Science, University of California Press.

Brown, K. T. & Murakami, M. (1964) A new receptor of the monkey retina with no detectable latency. *Nature* (London), **201**, 626–628.

Brown, K. T. & Tasaki, K. (1961) Localisation of electrical activity in the cat retina by an electrode marking method. *Journal of Physiology*, **158**, 281–295.

Cobb, W. A. & Morton, H. B. (1954) A new component of the human electroretinogram. *Journal of Physiology*. **123**, 36–37.

Cone, R. A. & Brown, P. K. (1967) Dependence of the early receptor potential on the orientation of rhodopsin. *Science*, **156**, 536.

Dewar, J. & McKendrick, J. G. (1873) On the physiological action of light. *Transactions of the Royal Society of Edinburgh*. **27**, 141–166.

Du Bois Reymond, E. (1849) *Untersuchungen über thierische Elektricitat*. pp. 256–257. Berlin: Reimer.

Einthoven, W. & Jolly, W. A. (1908) The form and magnitude of the electrical response of the eye to stimulation by light at various intensities. *Quarterly Journal of Experimental Physiology*. **1**, 373–416.

Francois, J., De Rouck, A., Cambie, E. & Zanen, A. (1974) In *L'Electrodiagnostic Des Affections Retiniennes*, Premier partie. pp. 20–33. Paris: Masson & Cie.

Frohlich, F. W. (1914) Beitrage zur allgemeinen Physiologie der Sinnesorgane. *Zeitschrift für Psychologie und Physiologie der Sinnesorgane. II. Abteil Sinnesphysiologie*, **48**, 28–164.

Gotch, F. (1903) The time relations of the photoelectric changes in the eyeball of the frog. *Journal of Physiology*, **29**, 388–410.

Granit, R. (1933) The components of the retinal action potential in mammals and their relation to the discharge in the optic nerves. *Journal of Physiology*, **77**, 207–239.

Granit, R. (1947) *Sensory Mechanisms of the Retina*. London: Oxford University Press.

Hartline, H. K. (1925) The electrical response to illumination of the eye in intact animals, including the human subject, and in decerebrate preparations. *American Journal of Physiology*, **121**, 400–415.

Holmgren, F. (1865) Method att objectivera effecten av ljusintryck pa retina. *Upsala Laekarefoerenings Foerhandlingar*, **1**, 177–191.

Karpe, G. (1945) The basis of clinical electroretinography. *Acta Ophthalmologica (København)*, Supp. 24.

Karpe, G. Rickenbach, K. & Thomasson, S. (1950) The clinical electroretinogram. I. The normal electroretinogram above fifty years of age. *Acta Ophthalmologica (København)*, **28**, 301–305.

Kojima, M. & Zrenner, E. (1978) Off-components in response to brief light flashes in the oscillatory potential of the human retinogram. *Albrecht von Graefes Archiv fur klinische und experimentelle Ophthalmologie*, **206**, 107–120.

Miller, R. F. & Dowling, J. E. (1970) Intracellular responses of the Müller cells of mudpuppy retina: their relation to 'b' wave of the electroretinogram. *Journal of Neurophysiology*, **33**, 323–341.

Noell, W. K. (1954) The origin of the electroretinogram. *American Journal of Ophthalmology*, **38**, 78–90.

Penn, R. D. & Hagins, W. A. (1972) Kinetics of the photocurrent of retinal rods. *Biophysical Journal*, **12**, 1073.

Riggs, L. A. (1941) Continuous and reproducable records of the electrical activity of the human retina. *Proceedings of the Society of Experimental Biology and Medicine*, **48**, 204.

Sachs, E. (1929) Die Aktionsströme Des menschlichen Auges, ihre Beziehung zu Reiz und Empfindung. *Klinische Wochenschrift*, **8**, 136–137.

Steinberg, R. H. (1966) Oscillatory activity in the optic tract of the cat. *Journal of Neurophysiology*, **29**, 139–156.

Wachtmeister, L. M. B. & Dowling, J. E. (1977) Microelectrode depth study of the oscillatory potentials of the electro-retinogram of the vertebrate retina. *Investigative Ophthalmology* (ARVO Supp.), **16**, 44.

Whitten, D. N. & Brown, K. T. (1973) The time courses of late receptor potentials from monkey cones and rods. *Vision Research*, **13**, 107–135.

CHAPTER THREE

The Electro-Oculogram

In the previous chapter we have been considering the electrical responses which are produced by exposing the eye to a brief flash of light. Although a variety of light stimuli are used in electroretinography they are all relatively short flashes lasting for milliseconds rather than seconds. The electro-oculogram is a slightly different technique which enables us to measure the electrical response of the eye to a prolonged light stimulus lasting several minutes.

It is important to remember that there is a difference in potential between the cornea and the posterior pole of the eye known as the corneo-retinal potential or the resting potential. It normally amounts to several millivolts, but is of course modified to form the electroretinogram when the eye is exposed to a brief flash. Unfortunately it is not easy to measure the corneo-retinal potential over long periods of time because in practice the steady response is obscured by blinks, random eye movements, and other artefacts. This problem can be resolved when performing electroretinography by using an AC coupled amplifier. This type of amplifier only responds to relatively rapid changes in potential and a steady base line is more easily maintained. When the eye is exposed to a continuous light stimulus a slow change in the corneo-retinal potential occurs. This would not normally be seen using an AC coupled amplifier, and the base line would be too unsteady to obtain accurate measurements if a directly coupled amplifier were used.

The electro-oculogram is a recording technique which allows an AC amplifier to be used to record these slow changes in the corneo-retinal potential; rapid changes of potential are produced by moving the eyes to and fro, and are fed through an AC amplifier to a pen recorder. These changes in potential have been shown to be related to the size of the corneo-retinal potential if the size of the eye movements is kept constant.

In order to perform the test, electrodes are placed on the skin on either side of the eye at the medial and the lateral canthi, and one indifferent electrode is usually placed on the forehead. The subject is seated facing a screen which can be illuminated. In addition two small red fixation lights are mounted on either side of the screen. The subject is then asked to look briskly from one fixation light to the other, thus making horizontal eye movements of a constant size.

The eye can be regarded as an electrical dipole, the cornea being positive with respect to the posterior pole. It can be seen from the diagram (Figure 3.1), how eye movements in a horizontal direction can produce a modified square wave and how the vertical limbs of this waveform can increase and decrease in size depending on the size of the corneo-retinal potential. The same method can of course be used to measure eye movements, but here we are concerned with changes in the corneo-retinal potential and the eye movements are kept at a constant value.

As long ago as 1929 it was shown that eye movements produce electrical changes which can be measured by skin electrodes (Meyers, 1929), but at that time it was assumed that these electrical changes were related to muscle action potentials. However, it was later conclusively proved that the changes in potential were due solely to the existence of the standing potential (Mowrer, Ruch and Miller, 1936). Furthermore, it was subsequently shown that the potential change exhibited by electro-oculography is directly proportional to the sine of the angle of rotation of the globe (Fenn and Hursh, 1937).

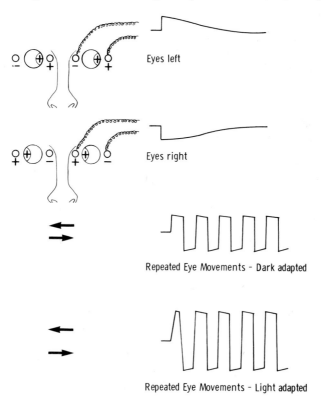

Figure 3.1. Diagram to illustrate the electrical response produced by eye movements and the influence of the corneo-retinal potential on this response.

Until the 1950s electro-oculography was used solely as a method of measuring eye movements and the earliest accounts of its use as a test of retinal function are those of Francois, Verriest and De Rouck (1955), and Ten Doesschate and Ten Doesschate (1956).

Electro-oculography thus provides a means of monitoring long-term changes in the corneo-retinal potential and in particular a means of assessing the changes induced by light. The tests devised by Francois, Verriest and De Rouck, and Arden and Kelsey are discussed in a later chapter, but at this stage it is necessary to describe the slightly unexpected behaviour of the corneo-retinal potential when the eye is exposed to a prolonged light stimulus.

First of all if the subject is placed in the dark, the corneo-retinal potential tends to fall in value to reach a minimal value. In continued darkness the potential remains at this low level but tends to wander up and down slightly. If a light stimulus is applied at this point, there is an initial electroretinographic response and then the potential falls for about two minutes after which it begins to rise steadily over a period of several minutes (Helig, Thaler and Scheiber, 1977). The initial fall has been termed 'the transient' and the rise has become known as 'the light rise'. After about seven minutes the corneo-retinal potential reaches a peak value and then begins to fall in spite of the fact that the light stimulus is still being applied. This fall of potential is followed by a further rise and it becomes apparent that the response has the form of a damped oscillation (Kris, 1958).

If the lights are switched off, the corneo-retinal potential falls back to the dark trough. A small positive peak can sometimes be seen immediately the lights are switched off, which corresponds with the negative transient at the beginning of the light rise (Figure 3.2). If a dim light stimulus is used a steady state may be rapidly reached after only two or three oscillations, but with brighter lights the oscillations may continue for a much longer period. It is important to realise that this technique does not directly measure the value of the corneo-retinal potential in millivolts, and readings are made in arbitrary units. In addition we cannot necessarily assume that the measured values are linearly related to the corneo-retinal potential. In practice the most reliable clinical assessment can be achieved by making a ratio of the light peak and dark trough. The clinical test is described in more detail in Chapter 7. It has now become customary to refer to the result of the test, rather than the technique itself, as the 'electro-oculogram'. Hence one may refer to a normal 'electro-oculogram' although the term can also be used to describe a method of measuring eye movements.

ORIGIN OF THE ELECTRO-OCULOGRAM AND ITS RELATION TO THE ELECTRORETINOGRAM

The electro-oculogram recorded with skin electrodes is probably the resultant of several potentials. Potentials in the skin or other parts of the body do not change as the eye rotates and therefore do not affect the results. Potentials arising in the eye itself, on the other hand, could be more important. For example, the cornea is thought to be polarised so that its anterior surface is negative, that is to say it acts against the resting potential. If the corneal potential were to be abolished then one might expect a corresponding increase

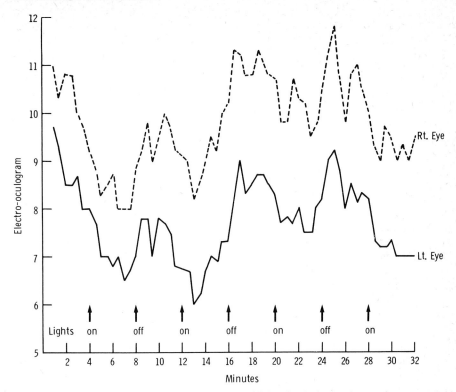

Figure 3.2. Experiment to show the effect of repeated light stimulation on the transient response.

in the resting potential. It is therefore interesting to find a considerable increase in the resting potential when the cornea is anaesthetised (Figure 3.3) (Arden and Fojas, 1962).

It is known that the standing potential, and also the value of the dark trough of the electro-oculogram, are markedly reduced by the administration of azide. This substance is known to produce selective damage to the pigment epithelium. Hence this may be the site of origin of at least part of the electro-oculographic response. But the light rise is markedly impaired by occlusion of the central retinal artery, both in man and in experimental animals, and one might expect the response to be spared if it arose solely from the pigment epithelium. There is also some evidence that the absorption spectrum of the electro-oculogram matches that of visual purple (Arden and Kelsey, 1962). On the other hand, in a more recent investigation blue and red lights were chosen to evoke equally large increases in the amplitude of the electro-oculogram. It was found that in five totally colour-blind subjects the response to red light was below normal, whereas the response to blue light was within the normal range. These results suggest that both the rods and the cones contribute to the normal electro-oculogram (Elenius and Aantas, 1973). The time course of the rise in value of the standing potential in response to light suggests that it may be reflecting the chemical process of light adaptation. Perhaps the slow rise of the corneo-retinal potential over seven minutes is a

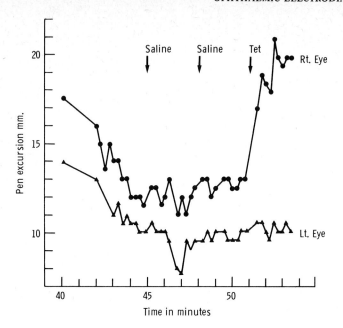

Figure 3.3. The effect of locally administered tetracaine on the corneo-retinal potential. Reproduced from Arden & Fojas (1962), *Archives of Ophthalmology*, **68**, 379. Copyright 1962, American Medical Association, with permission.

manifestation of the regeneration of photopigment. It has been suggested that the electro-oculogram is composed of two parts, a light-sensitive component arising in the receptors or perhaps more deeply in the retina, and a light-insensitive component arising in the pigment epithelium (Gouras, 1969).

Whereas it is possible to detect differences in the shape and size of the electroretinogram in the light-adapted and the dark-adapted state, it has not so far been possible to demonstrate photopic and scotopic responses using the electro-oculogram, although spectral sensitivity measurements have indicated a predominantly rod response with some evidence of cone activity (Elenius and Karo, 1966). In spite of all the differences in origin and behaviour between the electro-oculogram and the electroretinogram, pathological processes in the eye which cause alterations in one tend to cause similar changes in the other. This is probably because it is unusual for a disease process to be limited to one single layer of the retina. For example, a marked impairment of both the electro-oculogram and the electroretinogram is seen at an early stage in eyes suffering from retinitis pigmentosa. Claims have been made that in some instances either one or the other of these techniques show the first changes, but this may depend on the accuracy of the particular equipment used rather than the test itself. It has been claimed that in certain diseases the electro-retinogram may be normal when the electro-oculogram is grossly abnormal or vice versa, and this may be of diagnostic value. Patients with vitelliform macular degeneration, for example, may have a diminished light rise and a normal electroretinogram. It has also been shown that it may be possible to distinguish between a congenital retinal dysgenesis and a congenital retinal abiotrophy by the fact that in the former instance the electro-oculogram is normal, whereas both the electroretinogram and the electro-oculogram are affected in a congenital retinal abiotrophy (Henkes and Verduin, 1963).

Although there are one or two instances where the changes in the electro-oculogram do not reflect changes in the electroretinogram and vice versa, our knowledge of the meaning of these differences is still inadequate. In practice the important differences between these two tests may be summarised as follows:

1. The electroretinogram measures rapid changes in the resting potential in response to light, whereas the electro-oculogram measures slow changes.
2. A contact lens is not required for electro-oculography.
3. Less skill is required for electro-oculography and the equipment is more portable.
4. The electro-oculogram cannot easily be performed on patients who cannot fixate, and it is not very suitable for testing retinal function in blind patients.

PHYSIOLOGICAL VARIATIONS IN THE ELECTRO-OCULOGRAM

One of the problems which has beset the clinical use of the electro-oculogram is the variation in the response not only between individuals, but in one individual at different times (Kelsey, 1967). Van Lith and Balik made an extensive study of 15 normal subjects; the mean value of the Arden Index (the ratio of the light rise and dark trough) obtained from 140 experiments was 2·15 with a standard deviation of 0·25. They conclude that an index of less than 1·65 is highly likely to be abnormal if only one reading is taken. Values between 1·65 and 1·90 are borderline cases. In any given individual an alteration of more than 0·25 is suspicious and an alteration of more than 0·50 is likely to be pathological (Van Lith and Balik, 1970).

INTERFERENCE BETWEEN THE TWO EYES

There is little doubt that the electro-oculogram recorded from one eye is slightly modified by that from the other under certain circumstances. For example, when the light rise is abolished unilaterally, a paradoxical response is sometimes seen where a fall in amplitude occurs after the lights are switched on. This 'light fall' which is typically seen in the affected eye of patients with unilateral retinal detachment is thought to be due to spread of electrical changes from the sound eye.

REFERENCES

Arden, G. B. & Fojas, M. R. (1962) Electrophysiological abnormalities in pigmentary degenerations of the retina. *Archives of Ophthalmology*, **68**, 369–389.

Arden, G. B. & Kelsey, J. H. (1962) Changes produced by light in the standing potential of the human eye. *Journal of Physiology*, **161**, 189–204.

Elenius, V. & Aantaa, E. (1973) Light-induced increase in amplitude of the electro-oculogram; evoked with blue and red light in totally color-blind and normal humans. *Archives of Ophthalmology*, **90**, 60–63.

Elenius, V. & Karo, T. (1966) Cone activity in the light-induced response of the human electro-oculogram. *Pflügers Archiv für die gesamte Physiologie des Menschen und der Tiere*, **291**, 241–248.

Fenn, W. & Hursh, J. B. (1937) Movements of the eye when the lids are closed. *American Journal of Physiology*, **118**, 8–14.

Francois, J., Verriest, G. & De Rouck, A. (1955) Modification of the amplitude of the human electro-oculogram by light and dark adaptation. *British Journal of Ophthalmology*, **39**, 398–408.

Gouras, P. (1969) In *The Retina; Morphology, Function and Clinical Characteristics*, (Eds.) Straatsma, B., Hull, M., Alba, R. & Crescitelli, F. *UCLA Forum in Medical Sciences*, **8**, 865. Los Angeles: University of California Press.

Helig, P., Thaler, A. & Scheiber, V. (1977) The initial phase of the EOG oscillation. *Documenta Ophthalmologica* (Proceedings Series), **15**, 149–150.

Henkes, H. E. & Verduin, P. C. (1963) Dysgenesis or abiotrophy? A differentiation with the help of the electroretinogram and the electro-oculogram in Leber's congenital amaurosis. *Ophthalmologica*, **145**, 144–160.

Kelsey, J. H. (1967) Variations in the normal electro-oculogram. *British Journal of Ophthalmology*, **51**, 44–49.

Kris, C. (1958) Corneo-fundal potential changes during light and dark adaptation. *Nature*, **182**, 1027–1028.

Meyers, I. L. (1929) Electronystagmography. A graphic study of the active currents in nystagmus. *Archives of Neurology and Psychiatry*, **21**, 901.

Mowrer, O. H., Ruch, T. C. & Miller, N. E. (1936) The corneo-retinal potential difference as the basis of the galvanometric method of recording eye movements. *American Journal of Physiology*, **114**, 423–428.

Ten Doesschate, G. & Ten Doesschate, J. (1956) The influence of the state of adaptation on the resting potential of the human eye. *Ophthalmologica*, **132**, 308–320.

Van Lith, G. & Balik, J. (1970) Variability of the electro-oculogram. *Acta Ophthalmologica* (København), **48**, 1091–1096.

CHAPTER FOUR

The Visually Evoked Potential

The recording of the spontaneous electrical activity of the brain from electrodes placed on the scalp has been practised as a clinical routine for many years. Only over the past twenty years has it become possible to record the electrical changes over the scalp evoked by peripheral stimuli. The visually evoked potential is one of several evoked potentials which can be recorded from scalp electrodes. Such electrical changes can be produced by sound, by smell and taste, as well as by sensory stimulation. The changes evoked by visual stimuli were recorded in animals directly from the surface of the pia mater in the 1930s (Fischer, 1932). At that time it was well recognised that the alpha rhythm seen on normal electro-encephalographic traces could be accentuated by exposing the eyes to a light flashing at a similar frequency. When the eyes were exposed to repeated flashes at a different frequency, the electrical changes recorded from scalp electrodes became small and more or less lost against the background of the normal spontaneous activity of the brain.

Signal Averaging. The problem of detecting these small electrical signals was largely solved by the introduction of the technique of averaging. Before the development of modern electronics this simply entailed the superimposition of the repeated responses after each flash stimulus. Examining the trace after a single flash revealed little or no sign of any waveform that one might relate to the flash, but when a sufficient number of traces had been superimposed, a response could be discerned which was not visible on the single record. This method of mechanical averaging has now been supplanted by electronic averaging. The response following each consecutive stimulus is stored in the memory of a computer, and the average can be automatically displayed as a single trace on the face of an oscilloscope at the end of the operation. Figure 4.1 shows the effect of averaging on a raw EEG tracing obtained when the eyes were exposed to repeated light flashes.

If the responses to a large number of similar visual stimuli are averaged, the

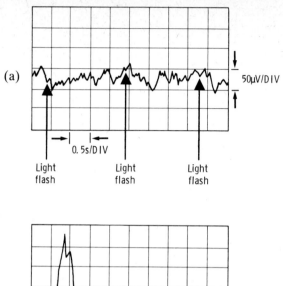

Figure 4.1. The effect of averaging. (a) EEG recorded with scalp electrodes during repeated light flashes of 1 msec duration at approximately 2-second intervals. Responses to the light flashes are buried by the EEG and by noise. (b) The same waveform after analysis by a signal-averaging instrument triggered from the light flash. A 25-microvolt response can be clearly detected after averaging with 256 sweeps. Note the difference in voltage amplitude scale for the two traces.

discrimination from irrelevant cortical activity can be improved greatly. From the clinical viewpoint the introduction of averaging was an important break-through, because we can now record visually evoked potentials (VEPs) as small as two or three microvolts. Furthermore, the nature of the response and its amplitude and waveform can be related to the type of visual stimulus in a way never before possible. As will be seen later, the development of the VEP offers the possibility of a true objective measure of visual acuity and of the visual field.

From the time of the early recordings of the average evoked potentials (Calvet et al, 1956; Ciganek, 1961) to the present day, there has been a gradual increase in the research interest in this subject. The research possibilities have attracted the attention of neurologists, psychiatrists, psychologists, physicists, and engineers, as well as opticians and ophthalmologists.

Method of Recording the Visually Evoked Potential

Many electrodiagnostic clinics throughout the world now investigate the VEP as a routine procedure, but because it is still in the stage of development no successful attempts at standardisation of the equipment have so far been made. By and large the equipment and electrodes do not differ greatly, but the type of stimulus used in different clinics varies considerably. The nature of the response recorded from the scalp may vary widely from clinic to clinic and records must be interpreted with great care.

In order to record the VEP, four groups of equipment are needed: a repeated visual stimulus is required; electrical contact with the patient's scalp must be achieved by means of suitable electrodes; electrical changes in these electrodes must be magnified by means of a suitable system of amplifiers; and an averaging computer and read-out system is needed to display the information obtained.

1. *The Stimulus*. This can be a diffuse flash of light or a pattern displayed on a screen. The diffuse flash or unstructured stimulus may of course vary in frequency intensity, size, or colour. The patterned stimulus is most popularly a checkerboard of black and white squares, although for some purposes lined gratings or other patterns are used. It is important to distinguish between pattern reversal and pattern appearance, because each produces a different

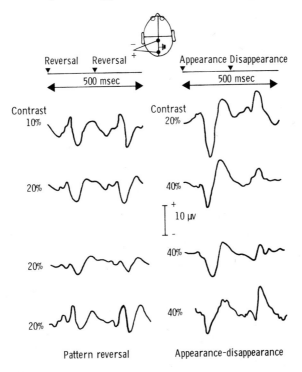

Figure 4.2. The response of four different subjects to pattern reversal (first column), and pattern appearance (second column). The totally different character of the trace produced by the two types of stimulus is seen. (After Spekreijse et al, 1973.)

response from the scalp. In the case of pattern reversal the luminosity of the black and white squares is reversed alternately, the black becoming white and the white becoming black. In the case of pattern appearance a black and white checkerboard is presented in an on-off sequence. It is also important to distinguish between a rapidly repeated stimulus and a slowly repeated stimulus for the same reasons. The rapidly repeated stimulus produces a sinusoidal type of response referred to as the 'steady state' response. Stimuli repeated less than two or three times a second produce a characteristic waveform known as the 'transient response' (see Figure 4.2 for examples of different types of response from different stimuli).

2. *The Electrodes*. Ideally the skin electrodes must make good contact, be electrically inert, and have a low electrical resistance. The most popular ones are made of silver coated with silver chloride, a layer of electrode jelly being placed between the electrode and the scalp. It may be held in place by collodion or a head strap. Fitting the scalp electrodes takes time and patience and should be performed by an experienced technician for best results. The exact positioning of the electrodes is critical. The standard 'ten-twenty' system of electro-encephalographers provides a useful variety of positions (see Figure 4.3), although some prefer to state their electrode positions as direct measurements from the inion. In practice the choice of electrode position depends upon the particular aspect of the VEP being investigated.

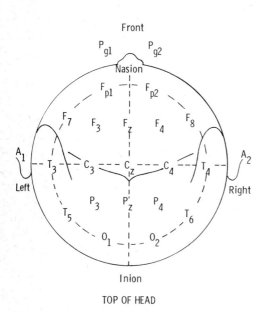

Figure 4.3. Standard international (10–20) electrode placement.

3. *The System of Amplifiers*. Usually two amplifiers are used, a preamplifier and a main amplifier, the system being designed to amplify the minute electrical signals from the scalp to a level acceptable for the computer and readout display. This must be done without causing undue distortion of the signal and without danger to the patient.

4. *The Averaging Computer and Read-out System*. The design and function of electronic equipment are continually being improved. Whereas until recently a small computer designed only for signal averaging was used, it is now more common to find larger and more versatile computers in use. These

(a)

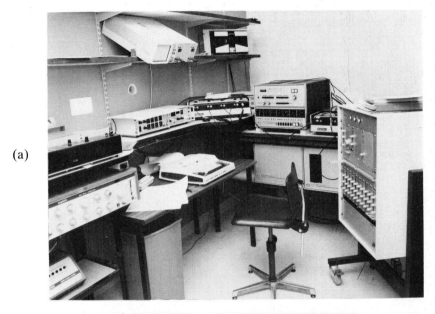

(b)

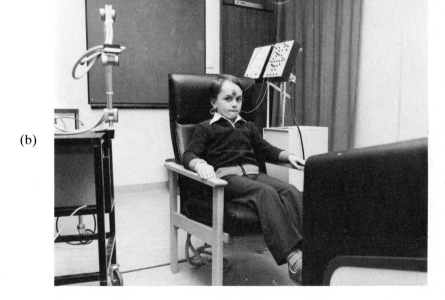

Figure 4.4. (a) Layout of main amplifiers, computer and read-out system in the electrodiagnostic clinic. (b) Testing room of the clinic showing patient seated with electrodes in position for recording the visually evoked potential.

allow the waveform of the response to be processed mathematically in a short space of time and provide a convenient way of storing records. Figure 4.4 shows a typical VEP recording system.

The Normal VEP

The character of the normal VEP depends upon the type of stimulus being used and the position on the scalp from which it is being recorded. It also varies greatly from one individual to another. In spite of these difficulties, reliable features, particularly of the transient response to a checkerboard stimulus, are beginning to be identified. Figure 4.5 shows the features of the response to a flash stimulus recorded from midline electrodes above the inion. The response to a pattern appearance stimulus is shown alongside it for comparison.

In general, three peaks are distinguishable on all these recordings; an initial positive peak at about 70–100 msec, a negative peak at about 100–130 msec and a second positive peak at about 150–200 msec. This last positive peak is often prominent in pattern stimulus records and is especially sensitive to changes in contrast and is favoured by binocular stimulation. (Spekreijse, Van der Tweel and Suidema, 1973). The timing of the peaks depends on the exact nature of the stimulus and also the position of the scalp electrodes (Allison et al, 1977). The response to a plain flash stimulus is smaller and less well defined and cannot easily be compared with the patterned response, although as the check size of a patterned stimulus becomes very large or very small, the electrical response more closely resembles that produced by an unstructured flash stimulus (see Figure 4.5).

The normal VEP has now been studied under a wide variety of stimulus conditions. Investigations of the effect of altering the size of the stimulus indicate that most of the response is derived from the central macula area of the retina (Regan, 1972). The VEP shows a progressive increase in size with

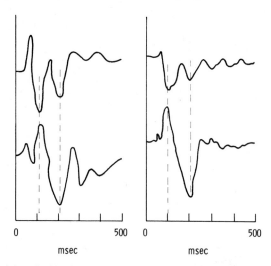

Figure 4.5. Potential evoked by flash presentation of a checkerboard pattern (lower trace) and a blank stimulus field (upper trace), for two subjects. (After Rietveld et al, 1967.)

dark adaptation and it is abolished by pressure blinding the exposed eye, recovering after about ninety seconds (Blake and Fox, 1973).

Many other types of stimulus have been used, and studies have been made on the effect of altering contours and the size of pattern elements, the effect of eccentricity of retinal stimulation, and the effect of retinal disparity in binocular stimulation (Harter, Seiple and Salmon, 1973; Cobb, Ettlinger and Morton, 1967).

The effect of age on the VEP has been extensively examined, and the possible value of this type of test in the investigation of the vision of young children has produced many studies in infants. It appears that the pattern-reversal VEP resembles that of an adult at the age of six months (Sokol and Dobson, 1976; Watanabe, Iwase and Hara, 1973; Harter, Deaton and Vernon Odom, 1977; Novikova and Filchikova, 1977; and Dustman, Schenkenberg and Beck, 1976). In premature infants the VEP is limited to the occipital region and gradually spreads with increasing age. The waveform also changes, and it has been claimed that the diffuse flash VEP of the premature infant can be distinguished from that of the full-term infant (Regan, 1972).

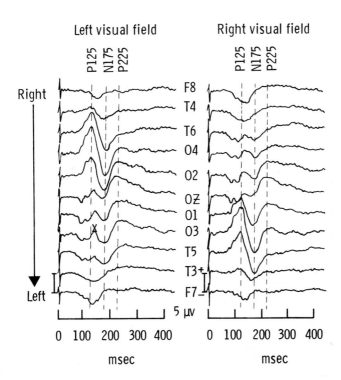

Figure 4.6. The VEP to pattern onset. Note that here stimulation of the left half-field produces a larger response over the right side of the scalp (Shagass et al, 1976).

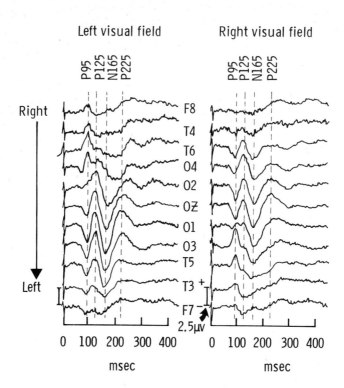

Figure 4.7. The VEP to pattern-reversal stimuli applied to right and left hemifields. Note that stimulation of the left half-field paradoxically appears to produce a larger response over the left side of the scalp and vice versa (Shagass et al, 1976).

The Visually Evoked Potential and the Visual Field

If different parts of the visual field are stimulated by a small patterned stimulus and the VEP measured from midline electrodes, the amount of information obtained is disappointing. This is not only because the response becomes very small when the stimulus is only a few degrees from fixation, but also because the method is not capable of detecting quite extensive defects in the visual field. Responses from the upper part of the field are always smaller than those from the lower part in normal subjects, using midline electrodes. Furthermore, all three components of the transient response show a polarity reversal when the stimulus is changed from upper to lower half (Halliday and Michael, 1970; Jeffreys, 1971). The information obtainable from a single midline electrode when different parts of the visual field are stimulated is therefore limited, and numerous workers are now investigating the detailed scalp topography of the response.

A more fruitful approach to the problem of relating the effect of stimulating different parts of the retina to the cortical evoked response has been gained from hemifield stimulation. By stimulating corresponding right or left half fields of vision and thereby presumably stimulating contralateral hemispheres, significant electrical changes can be measured from electrodes placed away from the midline on either side (Cobb and Morton, 1970; Lesevre and Remond, 1972). At first sight the results from these and other workers appear to conflict with one another: some claim clear-cut contralateral responses with half-field stimulation; others claim, surprisingly, a large response over the ipsilateral hemisphere. The apparent difference in these results is probably due to the different types of stimulus used, whether pattern reversal or pattern onset, and also to the fact that different peaks on the transient response were being measured. Thus an early peak, measured 90 msec after the stimulus, is found contralaterally and well away from the midline with pattern-onset stimulation, and a well-developed peak at 125 msec is found over the ipsilateral hemisphere with a pattern-reversal stimulus. (Figures 4.6 and 4.7 show more detailed results of this kind of work.) It can be seen that in the case of the pattern-reversal responses the positive peak at 125 msec is largely ipsilateral, as is the negative peak at 165 msec. The peak at 225 msec is largest in the midline in both pattern-onset and pattern-reversal stimulation, but the P125 is *contra*lateral with pattern-*onset* stimulation (Shagass, Amadeo and Roemer, 1976; Kriss and Halliday, 1980).

The VEP and the Measurement of Visual Acuity

The fact that blurring the outline of a checkerboard stimulus or altering its size can greatly influence the latency and the amplitude of the VEP has led to attempts to use the test to measure visual acuity. The results of such tests are not likely to have much meaning when compared with the results of standard Snellen test types because a different aspect of visual acuity is being measured in each case (see Figure 4.8 for effect of check size on the response). Psychophysical measurements of ability to detect changes in contrast can also be made and compared with the VEP using contrast gratings. Here the results of psychophysical testing can be more closely related to electrophysiological findings (Riggs, 1977).

The VEP has also been used in attempts to make an objective assessment of refractive error. Regan (1973) has shown that by rotating a stenopaeic slit in front of the cornea of a subject viewing a checkerboard stimulus, the axes of astigmatism can be determined. Once these axes have been ascertained, the necessary lens power in each axis can be determined by a variable-power lens system. A graph of VEP amplitude versus slit angle and another of VEP amplitude versus lens power can be produced electronically within a few seconds of starting the tests (see Figure 4.9).

The investigation of the electrical changes over the scalp has attracted the interest of research workers from many disciplines all over the world because such electrical changes might give some indication of the working of the brain itself. A rudimentary knowledge of the pattern of changes over the scalp in response to certain repeated stimuli is beginning to emerge. As the results in normal subjects are beginning to be understood more clearly, investigations into the changes in disease are also taking place. It will be shown later that the VEP has an important place in the detection of healed retrobulbar neur-

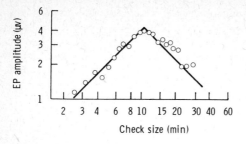

Figure 4.8. The effect of check size on the response. (Adapted from Regan, 1972.)

itis, and it is also used for assessing field defects in young children. Further examples of clinical application of the VEP will be considered in the appropriate chapters.

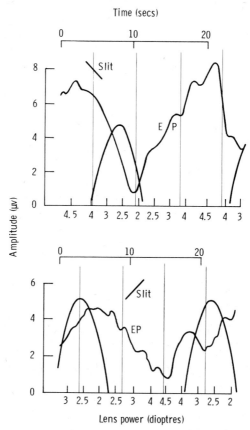

Figure 4.9. Upper and lower traces show relation of VEP amplitude to lens power for two different positions of a rotated slit. These types of result can be used to give an objective measurement of refractive error (Regan, 1973).

REFERENCES

Allison, T., Matsumiya, Y., Goff, G. D. & Goff, W. R. (1977) The scalp topography of the human VEP. *Electroencephalography and Clinical Neurophysiology (Montreal)*, **42**, 185.

Blake, R., & Fox, R. (1973) VER is abolished by pressure blinding and recorded largely 90 secs. after: Visually evoked cortical potentials during pressure blinding. *Vision Research*, **13**, 501.

Calvet, J., Cathala, H. P., Hirsch, J. & Scherrer, J. (1956) La réponse corticale visuelle de l'homme etudiée par une methode d'integration. *Comptes Rendus des Séances de la Société de Biologie et de Ses Filiales (Paris)*, **150**, 1348.

Ciganek, L. (1961) The electroencephalogram response to light stimulus (evoked potential) in man. *Electroencephalography and Clinical Neurophysiology* (Montreal), **13**, 165.

Cobb, W. A., Ettlinger, G. & Morton, H. B. (1967) Visual evoked potentials in binocular rivalry: *Electroencephalography and Clinical Neurophysiology (Montreal)*, **26**, 100.

Cobb, W. A. & Morton, H. B. (1970) Evoked potentials from the human scalp to visual half-field stimulation. *Journal of Physiology (London)*, **208**, 398–408.

Dustman, R. E., Schenkenberg, T. & Beck, E. C. (1976) The development of the evoked response as a diagnostic and evaluative procedure. In: *Developmental Psychophysiology of Mental Retardation*, Ed. Ratha Karrer. Springfield, Ill: Charles C. Thomas.

Fischer, M. H. (1932) VEP from pia mater. I. Elektrobiologische Erscheinungen an der Hirnrinde. *Pflügers Archiv für die gesamte Physiologie des Menschen und der Tiere*, **230**, 160.

Halliday, A. M. & Michael, W. F. (1970) Changes in pattern evoked responses in man associated with vertical and horizontal meridians of the visual field. *Journal of Physiology (London)*, **208**, 499.

Harter, M. R., Deaton, F. & Vernon Odom, J. (1977) Maturation of evoked potential and visual preference in 6–45 day old infants: effect of check size on visual acuity and refractive error. *Electroencephalography and Clinical Neurophysiology (Montreal)*, **42**, 595.

Harter, M. R., Seiple, W. H. & Salmon, L. (1973) Binocular summation of VER. *Vision Research*, **13**, 1433.

Jeffreys, D. A. (1971) Cortical source locations of pattern retarded VEP's recorded from human scalp. *Nature*, **229**, 502.

Kriss, A. & Halliday, A. M. (1980) Comparison of evoked potentials to pattern onset, offset and reversal by movement. In *Evoked Potentials: Proceedings of the International Symposium, Nottingham.* C. Barber (Ed). p. 205. Lancaster: M.T.P. Press.

Lesevre, N. & Remond, A. (1972) Potentials evoked by patterns: effect of pattern dimensions and contrast density. *Electroencephalography and Clinical Neurophysiology (Montreal)*, **32**, 593.

Novikova, L. A. & Filchikova, L. I. (1977) Influence of defocussing an optical stimulus on human VEP. *Zhurnal vȳssheĭ nervoĭ deyatel' nosti imeni P. Pavlova*, **27**, 98.

Regan, D. (1972) *Evoked Potentials*, pp. 109 and 190. London: Chapman and Hall.

Regan, D. (1973) Rapid objective refraction using evoked brain potentials. *Investigative Ophthalmology*, **12**, 669.

Riggs, L. A. (1977) In ERG, VER and Psychophysics. *Documenta Ophthalmologica* (Proceedings Series), **15**, 3–12.

Shagass, C., Amadeo, M., & Roemer, R. A. (1976) Optical distibution of potentials evoked by half-field pattern reversal and pattern onset stimuli. *Electroencephalography and Clinical Neurophysiology*, **41**, 609.

Sokol, S. & Dobson, V. (1976) Pattern reversal VER in infants. *Investigative Ophthalmology*, **15**, 58.

Spekreijse, H., Van der Tweel, L. H. & Suidema, Th. (1973) Contrast evoked responses in man. *Vision Research*, **13**, 1577.

Watanabe, K., Iwase, K. & Hara, K. (1973) VER during sleep and wakefulness in preterm infants. *Electroencephalography and Clinical Neurophysiology (Montreal)*, **34**, 571.

CHAPTER FIVE

Other Electrodiagnostic Techniques

The primary concern of this book is to consider the diagnostic value of the changes in bioelectric potential exhibited by the retina. Several other techniques are now being developed which entail making electrical measurements in and around the eye. Some of these techniques are concerned with the analysis of eye movements and some have so far only been used for research purposes. Before we proceed to consider the clinical applications of electro-retinography and electro-oculography in the next section of the book, it is appropriate to consider some of these related techniques.

ELECTRONYSTAGMOGRAPHY

The investigation of nystagmus is common ground for the opthalmologist and the otolaryngologist as well as the neurologist. Its study involves the accurate recording of eye movements and a variety of methods are available to achieve this. The simplest method is by corneal reflection. A light source is reflected from and focused by the cornea and a simple lens system onto moving light-sensitive paper. A more accurate method employs a photo-cell to detect changes in light reflection with eye movement. Both these methods have the disadvantage that they are not effective when the lids are closed or in darkness. This is an important deficiency because it is helpful to examine nystagmus both when the patient is fixing and when fixation is abolished by darkness or lid closure. Electronystagmography has the great advantage that it can measure eye movements under all these conditions; in particular, it has allowed the extensive studies of eye movements during sleep which have been made in recent years.

The principle of electronystagmography is identical with that of electro-oculography, although here one is not concerned with any changes in the corneo-retinal potential but only with the combined effect of a steady corneo-retinal potential and eye movements. Nystagmus produces a characteristic trace which can be analysed in detail. A neat method for doing this has been described which employs a DC amplifier. The base line is kept steady by incorporating a chopper amplifier as well, and by paying great attention to the preparation of the electrodes (Dix, Hallpike and Hood, 1963). The chopper amplifier effectively converts the DC signal into AC by chopping out bits of it at regular intervals so that a smooth DC signal becomes a square wave (Figure 5.1). This converted signal is then amplified and reconverted to DC. The whole exercise amounts to an electronic trick for maintaining a steady base line. In practice it means that sustained movements of the eyes to the right or left produce a corresponding and sustained movement of the pen recorder arm.

The clinical value of the method depends to some extent on the fact that nystagmus due to peripheral lesions of the eighth cranial nerve has different features from that due to central lesions. For example, nystagmus due to a peripheral nerve lesion tends to be abolished by fixation, but may reappear in darkness or when the lids are closed. Nystagmus can be measured after it has been induced or inhibited by a wide variety of stimuli such as watching a moving pendulum, rotating the patient, neck torsion, caloric and galvanic stimulation as well as other variations on a similar theme. Analysis of the electronystagmograms obtained by such methods may be useful in the diagnosis of disseminated sclerosis. A medico-legal application has also been found in investigating the nystagmus induced by alcohol (Greiner et al, 1971; Decroix, 1978).

ELECTROMYOGRAPHY

The recording of action potentials from motor units within muscle became possible with the invention of the concentric needle electrode (Adrian and Bronk, 1928). The needle contains an insulated core which may be single or double depending on the type of recording that is required. The spike potentials can be recorded with equipment similar to that required for electroretinography; they are very rapid and care should be taken that they are not wiped out by the high frequency cut-off of the amplifier. Recording is conveniently done on Polaroid film from the face of an oscilloscope. When the concentric needle has been inserted into the muscle, spikes appear when the muscle contracts. As the strength of contraction is increased the spike frequency increases up to 70 per second or more, and at the same time there is an increase in the number of motor units which produce the spikes. In the case

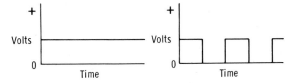

Figure 5.1. First stage in the treatment of a DC potential by a chopper amplifier. On the left, a continuous DC potential and on the right, the resulting square wave.

of peripheral nerve lesions, the number of firing units is reduced, and with lower motor neurone lesions spontaneous bursts of discharge may be evident. When the muscle itself is diseased, the number of firing motor units may be well preserved, but the duration of each unit discharge is shorter.

Examination of the spike discharges from the extra-ocular muscles requires the use of specially fine needles and extra skill is needed to insert the needles. The technique has been used to demonstrate the reciprocal innervation of opposing recti. It has also been shown that the levator palpebrae superioris is inhibited during the act of blinking. By and large there would appear to be a fundamental similarity between the responses obtained from extra-ocular muscles and those obtained from muscles elsewhere (Breinin, 1962).

Electromyography has now been used to investigate a wide variety of disorders of the extra-ocular muscles, but in most cases so far the clinical signs of the disorder are quite apparent by the time that the electromyogram becomes abnormal. Of special interest has been the investigations of Duane's syndrome where marked abnormalities have been found, the most important of these being an abnormality of the firing pattern of the lateral rectus. This may show paradoxical innervation or incomplete inhibition on adduction (Strachan and Brown, 1972). Interesting results have also been reported in abnormal regeneration of the third nerve, progressive ocular myopathy and myasthenia gravis. In myasthenia gravis the fatiguing phenomenon is evident as a reduction in the amplitude of the spikes with time.

ULTRASONOGRAPHY

Although ultrasonography involves the use of electronic equipment, it is not concerned with the measurement of the corneo-retinal potential or indeed of any bioelectric potential. Its use is said to have been born from the *Titanic*

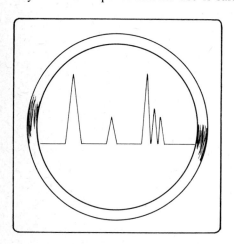

Figure 5.2. The type of trace seen in A-scan ultrasonography showing typical echo pulses.

tragedy as the result of an intensive search for methods of tracking icebergs. Pulses of high-frequency sound waves are transmitted into the eye and the echoes from the different surfaces are analysed. In ophthalmology frequencies of 2 to 4 MHz are used. Sound waves are produced and detected by electro-

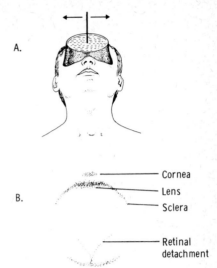

Figure 5.3 A. Position of the water bath and probe for B-scan ultrasonography. B. Type of trace seen on the face of the oscilloscope in B-scan ultrasonography.

acoustic transducers. These are devices for converting electricity into sound and vice versa; their working principle relies on the piezoelectric effect. Piezoelectric substances change size under the effect of an electric field and rapid changes of size produce sound waves. Piezoelectric substances also produce changes in an electric field if their size is changed. Thus sound vibrations can be converted into electrical changes.

In ophthalmic ultrasonography brief pulses of high frequency sound lasting less than one microsecond are pulsed into the eye and the received pulses are displayed on a cathode ray screen. Figure 5.2 is a diagram to illustrate A-scan ultrasonography. Pulses are reflected from all boundaries between different media and the larger the echo, the larger the pulse that is displayed on the screen. The vertical axis on the oscilloscope thus represents echo size whereas the horizontal axis represents time. The equipment for A-scan ultrasonography can be relatively simple; a pencil-like probe has a flattened end which is lubricated and placed on the anaesthetised cornea or sclera and echoes are seen immediately on the screen of the oscilloscope. These are then photographed.

B-scan ultrasonography is an important development of the A-scan technique. Here the beam of the oscilloscope is light modulated so that larger echoes appear brighter and not as larger pulses on the screen. In addition the transducer probe is moved around the surface of the eye in a controlled manner and the horizontal deflection of the cathode ray tube is synchronised with the motion of the transducer. The application of the probe is here a more complex operation; a sealed water bath is placed around the eyes and orbits and the probe is immersed in water. A storage oscilloscope tube is used so that a picture representing a cross-section of the eye is gradually built up on the screen (Figure 5.3).

In skilled hands ultrasound can be used to diagnose detachments in opaque media and to detect solid tumours within the eye. A-scan ultrasonography provides a way of making accurate *in vivo* measurements of the globe and its contents (Vanýsek, Preisova and Obraz, 1970).

B-scan ultrasonography is now finding an important place in the diagnosis of orbital lesions, and in many centres it is now part of the routine investigation of proptosis (Sutherland, 1978).

ELECTRICAL PHOSPHENES

The eye is not solely light sensitive, and other modalities can be used to produce the sensation of light. If an electric current is passed through the eye, patterns of light can be seen which depend on the type of current and electrode that are used. These are known as phosphenes. If the eye is temporarily blinded by applying pressure to it to occlude the circulation, then no phosphenes are seen, even if the current is increased to 150 times the threshold for the unblinded eye. This confirms that the phosphene arises within the eye itself and indicates that the retina must be much more sensitive to electrical stimulation than the optic nerve. Some interesting experiments have been carried out using these phosphenes; the eye does not adapt significantly to the brightness, the same strength of current being required for the light-adapted and the dark-adapted eye. Altering the shape and position of the phosphene and other experiments suggest that the site of stimulation is the bipolar layer or the inner segments of the rods and cones (Brindley, 1970a).

Phosphenes may also be produced by electrical stimulation of the occipital poles of the cerebral hemispheres. This fact was known to neurosurgeons many years ago but the idea of making use of it to construct a visual prosthetic device has only been put into practice recently (Brindley, 1970b). The signals arise from radio transmitters worn in a hat and are transmitted across the scalp to a large number of minute radio receivers implanted between the parietal bone and the pericranium. Cables from these receivers link up with electrodes implanted in the occipital cortex. Using this arrangement it is possible to enable a totally blind person to 'see' letters and even read. The number of patients chosen for this type of prosthesis has necessarily been limited, but the method seems to open up exciting prospects for the future.

THE OBJECTIVE MEASUREMENT OF VISUAL ACUITY

A large part of the ophthalmologist's time is spent in measuring visual acuity. This requires time and patience in elderly, confused or illiterate patients, and below the age of two or three, accurate testing of the visual acuity is not possible. For all these reasons an objective test would be a major advance in ophthalmic practice. Electrodiagnostic tests can at present provide two lines of approach, neither of which has been fully explored. Firstly, the visually evoked potential can be used as a crude test of visual acuity and this has already been discussed in the chapter devoted to that subject. Secondly, electronystagmography can be used to measure the optokinetic nystagmus induced by viewing a rotating striped drum. The diameter of the stripes is varied and a point arises at which they are so narrow that they cannot be discerned and no optokinetic nystagmus results (Wolin and Dillman, 1964; Lewkonia, 1969).

COMPUTER-ASSISTED TOMOGRAPHY

It would not be possible to end this brief account of electrodiagnostic techniques other than those measuring the corneo-retinal potential, without mentioning a revolutionary advance in radiology which has recently been introduced. Computer-assisted tomography was originally described at the Congress of the British Institute of Radiology (Ambrose and Hounsfield, 1972). A detailed account of the apparatus has been given by Hounsfield (1973) and its clinical application in the demonstration of intracranial space-occupying lesions by Ambrose (1973, 1974). Such clarity and detail of normal and abnormal anatomy can be obtained that the method is likely to supersede many other techniques. Unlike computer-assisted tomography, the visually evoked response, the electroretinogram and the electro-oculogram give a measure of the function rather than the morphology of the structure under investigation and these two kinds of test may complement one another in the future.

REFERENCES

Adrian, E. D. & Bronk, D. W. (1928) The discharges of impulses in motor nerve fibres. *Journal of Physiology*, **66**, 81–101.
Ambrose, J. (1973) Computerized transverse axial scanning (tomography): Part II. Clinical application. *British Journal of Radiology*, **46**, 1023–1047.
Ambrose, J. (1974) Computerized x-ray scanning of the brain. *Journal of Neurosurgery*, **40**, 679–695.
Ambrose, J. & Hounsfield, D. (1972) *Proceedings of the 32nd Annual Congress of the British Institute of Radiology*, Ch. 4.
Breinin, G. M. (1962) The electrophysiology of extra-ocular muscle. *American Ophthalmological Society*, **65**, 73.
Brindley, G. S. (1970a) In *Physiology of the Retina and Visual Pathway*. 2nd Edition, **6**, 155. *Monographs of the Physiological Society*. London: Edward Arnold.
Brindley, G. S. (1970b) Sensations produced by electrical stimulation of the occipital poles of the cerebral hemispheres and their use in constructing visual prostheses. *Annals of the Royal College of Surgeons of England*, **47**, 106–108.
Decroix, G. (1978) Electronystagmography. Proceedings of the 11th Symposium, Lille, 1977. *Rivista oto-neuro-oftalmologica*, **50**, 185–244.
Dix, M. R., Hallpike, C. S. & Hood, J. D. (1963) Electronystagmography and its uses in the study of spontaneous nystagmus. *Transactions of the Ophthalmological Society of the United Kingdom*, **83**, 531–536.
Greiner, G. F., Collard, M., Conraux, C. & Haushalter, G. (1971) Electronystagmographic changes induced by alcohol. *Rivista Oto-Neuro-Oftalmologica* (Bologna), **43**, 198–206.
Hounsfield, G. M. (1973) Computerized transverse axial scanning (tomography): Part I. Description of system. *British Journal of Radiology*, **46**, 1016–1022.
Lewkonia, I. (1969) Objective assessment of visual acuity by induction of optokinetic nystagmus. *British Journal of Ophthalmology*, **53**, 641–644.
Strachan, I. M. & Brown, B. H. (1972) Electromyography of extra-ocular muscles in Duane's syndrome. *British Journal of Ophthalmology*, **56**, 594.
Sutherland, G. R. (1978) The contribution of echography in the diagnosis of proptosis. *British Journal of Radiology*, **51**, 116–121.
Vanÿsek, J., Preisova, J. & Obraz, J. (1970) *Ultrasonography in Ophthalmology*. London: Butterworth.
Wolin, L. R. & Dillman, A. (1964) Objective measurement of visual acuity. *Archives of Ophthalmology*, **71**, 822–826.

PART TWO

Clinical Applications

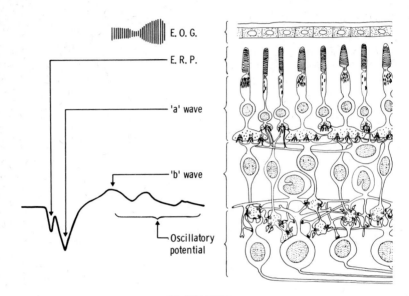

E. O. G.

E. R. P.

'a' wave

'b' wave

Oscillatory
potential

PLATE TWO

Origins of components of electrical response.

CHAPTER SIX

The Organisation of an Ophthalmic Electrodiagnostic Clinic

In the following pages it is proposed to consider some of the facts and, where possible, some of the figures relating to the establishment of a functioning electrodiagnostic clinic. For anyone with a particular interest in the subject it would be a mistake to be discouraged by the apparent high cost of such a project because it is possible, although not preferable, to practise electroretinography or electro-oculography on a shoestring. Many hospitals have an old EEG amplifier lying derelict in some dark corner, and in the absence of funds such equipment combined with an electrical penwriter can be adapted for these purposes. The amplifier and penwriter used in electrocardiography can also be adapted relatively simply for performing electro-oculograms. But although it is my purpose to encourage the enthusiast it is not my aim to advocate a second-best system, and we shall consider here the minimum requirements for a clinic to provide useful clinical information and to make full use of the latest advances in equipment design. In putting forward plans for such a clinic I visualise a small unit appropriate for a population of about one million. There are, of course, several large and highly organised ophthalmic electrodiagnostic units in existence, notably at Moorfields Eye Hospital, London, and also in Rotterdam, to mention only two.

Rapid advances are made in the design of electronic equipment from year to year and this causes difficulties when one is attempting to recommend a particular piece of equipment. Although specific items are mentioned here, they are usually mentioned because we ourselves have found them reliable and effective and they are given as a guide line only. Where possible an estimate of the cost of equipment has been given, but in these days of inflation these costs may be quite incorrect by the time this book is published. However, rather than omit them altogether it seemed that it might be helpful to present them as at 1979 values and the reader can adjust his sights accordingly.

PLANNING THE CLINIC

The initial step is to formulate a plan which can be presented to one's immediate colleagues, and at this stage it is advisable to consult with the nearest medical physics department and a hospital administrator. It is important to decide to what extent the clinic is to have a research function and to what extent it will deal with clinical problems. The answer to this question will decide whence the funds for the clinic are to be derived and which source is to be approached once the project has been approved by one's colleagues. If a more sophisticated computer is to be used, it is worth considering sharing it with the ear, nose and throat department, the neurology department, and the medical physics department. The clinic may have to be planned with this in mind. The whole conception might be considered under the following headings.

Site of the Clinic

A large room will be required which can be reached by patients in wheelchairs and which is preferably close to the main ophthalmic outpatient department. The minimum size should be about 15 metres×15 metres, but more space than this may be needed if visually evoked potentials are also being recorded. It is also convenient to have a separate room for reporting, especially if there is not a secretariat near at hand. It is advantageous to be able to perform general anaesthesia in the clinic, but if the anaesthetists are not happy about such an arrangement it will be necessary to convey the equipment on a trolley to the operating theatre. In either case it is useful if the clinic is not far removed from the ophthalmic operating theatre.

Electrical interference can be a major problem in the modern hospital, where there is inevitably a large amount of equipment which radiates noise at mains frequency. This can interfere with the base line of the trace, but there are also other sources of electrical noise, such as the local call system, the ambulance radio system, or even pneumatic drill compressors working in the road outside—the latter seem to be strangely attracted to hospitals. In practice, perhaps rather surprisingly, electrical noise is not usually a serious problem for electroretinography and electro-oculography and it is usually only necessary to site the room as far as possible from known sources. When the visually evoked potential is being recorded, considerably more amplification is required and the signal from the patient is much more likely to be obliterated by external interference. For these purposes it is preferable to work in a screened room. A copper cage provides the best screen for patient and equipment, although this makes the working atmosphere very claustrophobic and is also very expensive to erect. Many large clinics produce excellent results without screening and the decision to screen must depend on the likely level of local interference.

We have not experienced any difficulty in our own clinic without screening, but we have had some difficulty when the equipment has been transferred to the operating theatre to test children under general anaesthesia. On one occasion a team of nurses circulated through the hospital switching off all possible sources of interference when this was particularly troublesome in the theatre. A noise-free result was never obtained and a neglected refrigerator was accidentally defrosted.

Obviously a power supply is essential: at least three power points and preferably more should be available. A washbasin is also essential. It must be possible to make the room completely dark and for this reason a good ventilation system is necessary; a poor-quality electric fan may cause electrical interference. Strip lighting also causes some interference, but this does not seem to be a serious problem for routine clinical work since it is usually switched off when the measurements are made.

The Layout of the Clinic

It is convenient if the available space is divided into four separate but adjoining rooms (Figure 6.1). A recording room directly adjoins the clinic room and this is subdivided into an area for electroretinography and electro-oculography, and an area for performing visually evoked potentials. In the plan shown here it is suggested that a reporting room is included. This room would contain a desk, typewriter, coathangers, etc., as well as a shelf for reference books.

In the clinic room for electroretinography and electro-oculography a dental chair is positioned so that leads from the patient can be conveniently passed through the adjoining wall to the recording room. A cupboard containing electrode jelly, sterilising solutions, saline, plaster strapping, scissors and electrodes is needed, and a shelf or trolley should be available on which to lay up these items when they are in use. The stimulus lights and washbasin are placed in suitable positions in relation to the dental chair.

In the visually evoked potential part of the clinic room, more space is occupied by the stimulus light; a dental chair is also required here and leads

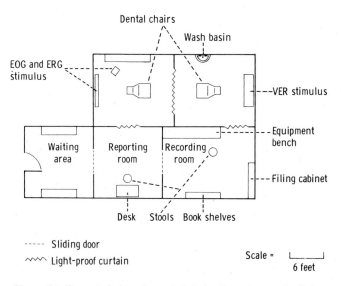

Figure 6.1. Suggested plan of an ophthalmic electrodiagnostic clinic.

pass from the patient to the recording room in a similar manner. This part of the clinic should house facilities for testing visual acuity and also a set of trial lenses.

The recording room contains a bench for the equipment which will include amplifiers, oscilloscope and averager and possibly other items, such as a pen-recorder or an X–Y plotter. A filing cabinet for records is best kept in here, as well as some essential tools such as screwdrivers, soldering iron and pliers.

Apart from the layout described, it may be necessary to have a waiting area for patients if the clinic is far removed from the main outpatient department. It is important to try to avoid leaving elderly patients in wheelchairs in draughty passages.

Figure 6.2 is a view of part of the clinic in Rotterdam. In one room a variety of tests can be performed. These include the visually evoked potential, electro-oculography and electroretinography, and in particular electro-oculography can be performed under general anaesthesia (see Chapter 7).

Obviously, the layout of the clinic must depend to a large extent on local circumstances. For example, it may be more convenient to associate the clinic with the department of electro-encephalography, or perhaps the medical physics department.

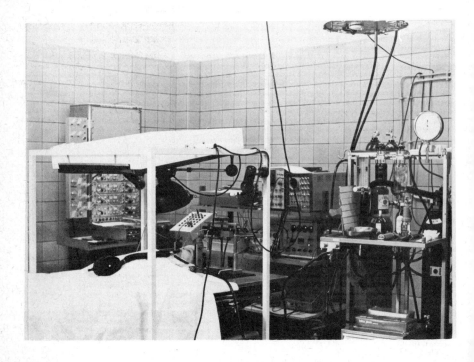

Figure 6.2. Some of the ophthalmic electrodiagnostic facilities at Rotterdam. (Reproduced by permission of Professor H. E. Henkes, Rotterdam.)

Equipment Required in the Clinic

Electroretinography

The stimulus light needs to be versatile if any clinical research is contemplated, but we have found that a photoflash gives the most useful type of response although it is not easy to calibrate. If the early receptor potential is to be elicited then a photoflash of about 25 J should be used. This type of flash tube produces a strong electrical artefact and it should be positioned at least one metre from the eye and screened as well as possible. The light-emitting side of the flash (which cannot of course be screened), must be directed into a light guide if sufficient light is to reach the eye. The light guide may be the fibre optic variety and this is very convenient, being fully flexible, or it may simply consist of a Perspex rod with a diameter of 2 cm. Needless to say, the Perspex rod is very much less expensive than the fibre optics light guide. Rapidly repeated flashes cannot be produced by a photoflash and it is therefore necessary to supplement this with a stroboscope of some kind. A commercial xenon strobe is quite suitable. It is necessary to be able to place filters in front of the stroboscope and the instrument may have to be adapted slightly for this purpose. It is quite feasible to stimulate both eyes simultaneously and apart from ensuring that both eyes are exposed to exactly the same stimulus strength, it is time saving. For this purpose a double Perspex tube or fibre optics light guide can be attached to the photoflash (Figure 6.3). Alternatively, a spectacle frame may be adapted to hold the ends of a light guide.

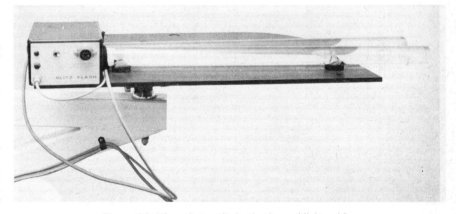

Figure 6.3. View of photoflash stimulus and light guide.

The skin electrodes must be chosen carefully since inadequate ones may increase the pick-up of electrical noise considerably. Standard electrodes as used for electrocardiography have been found effective, for example those made by Elema Schönander. It is an advantage if they have a lightproof and waterproof cover to them. The contact lens electrode is now available commercially (Figure 6.4). It will be seen in the next chapter that although a variety of lenses have been designed, variations in the type of lens do not seem to alter the response in a significant manner. There is an important exception to this, however; when recording the early receptor potential with

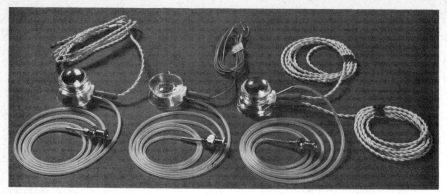

Figure 6.4. Three types of standard commercially available contact lens electrodes. (By courtesy of Keeler Ltd., London.)

a photoflash stimulus, a silver electrode cannot be incorporated in the lens because of the marked photo-electric effect of light on silver. The best material to use is malleable stainless steel or platinum, and it is safer to blacken the edges of the lens and the side arm to prevent light scatter. A type of lens incorporating these features is shown in Figure 6.5. The figure also shows a contact lens electrode designed in our clinic which uses carbon as the conducting medium, and a carbon fibre wire connection. This electrode has been especially easy to use and is artefact-free. Krakau and Öhman have described an electrode which is placed on the end of a Perspex rod and positioned in contact with the cornea under slit lamp control. A stimulus light is incorporated within the Perspex rod. Thus they introduced the idea that electroretinography should compare with applanation tonometry as an accessory function of the slit lamp microscope. (Krakau and Öhman 1975).

The wiring from connecting electrodes to the preamplifier must be light and well screened. The screening around the wire must be connected to earth, but one must be careful not to connect the screen at both ends of the wire to earth since this may produce what is known as an 'earth loop'. Under these circumstances the electrical noise may be greatly increased. Filotex is a high-quality type of screened wire which is suitable.

A preamplifier is now required, which enlarges the signal to a level at which it can be fed into an oscilloscope. The properties of such an amplifier should be as follows. Firstly, the amplifier must have a high input impedance (see glossary), with a common mode rejection of 90 to 100 dB. Secondly, it must have a frequency response of approximately 0.1 Hz to 5 Hz. If the upper limit of the frequency response is lowered to 300 Hz then an electroretinogram can still be recorded with a greatly reduced noise level. Unfortunately, this kind of 'top cut' eliminates the leading edge of the early receptor potential which is very rapid. Thirdly, the gain of the preamplifier should be ×1000. This means that the signal is boosted from 0.5 mV to 0.5 V and this size of signal is suitable for most oscilloscopes.

In recent years there has been concern over the safety of electromedical equipment, although this has been mainly limited to electrocardiography where there is a remote risk of affecting the cardiac rhythm by applying

(a)

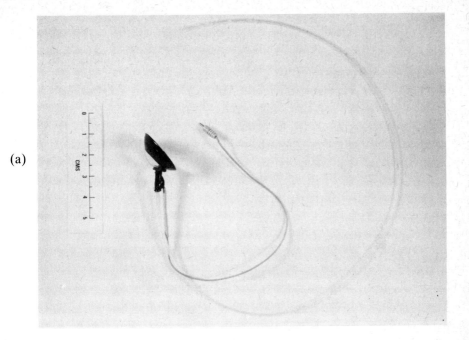

(b)

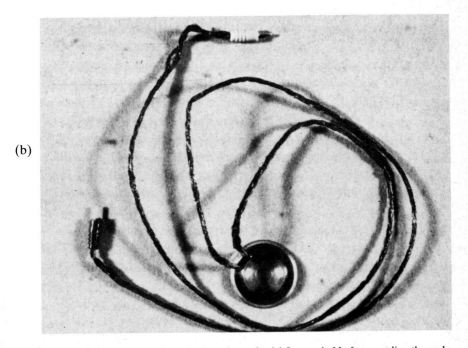

Figure 6.5. Two further types of contact lens electrode. (a) Lens suitable for recording the early receptor potential. (b) A carbon-carbon fibre lens electrode.

minute currents to the cardiac muscle. Although the risk of electrical injury to the eye from an amplifier with high input impedance must be minimal, it is likely that in the near future there will be legislation specifying that all pre-amplifiers must be of a special type known as isolated amplifiers. In these amplifiers the current flowing in the patients' leads is limited to a safe value. They have an additional advantage of good common mode rejection (see Glossary).

An isolated amplifier with the above characteristics is made by Analog Devices. A power supply is also required for this amplifier as an extra item.

Many oscilloscopes are available at the present time. Tektronix make a well-tried and popular series. Several different facilities are offered in the various models, but it is advisable to have a storage tube with a dual beam. Tektronix 5 100 series oscilloscope could be used. These instruments are provided with space for different plug-in units and a suitable unit for these purposes would be the amplifier 5A15.

Most oscilloscope manufacturers also can produce a camera which fits the face of the oscilloscope and the Tektronix instrument has a choice of two. The more expensive one is well worth having for its additional facilities.

We still have not mentioned all the equipment required for producing an electroretinogram because it is necessary to have a system for co-ordinating the stimulus flash, the camera and the beam of the oscilloscope. This system of 'triggering' is best done electronically and the equipment, which is relatively simple, can be most conveniently made up in a local workshop.

Electro-oculography

The equipment used can be the same as that used for electroretinography but the setting of the preamplifier is different, and the time base of the oscilloscope must be altered. The electrodes are also the same, although a contact lens is not required (Figure 6.6). The stimulus light is of course quite different and can be constructed from a bank of horizontally mounted strip lights covered by a diffusing screen and incorporating a red fixation light.

The gain of the preamplifier can be the same as that used for electro-retinography but the top cut can be much lower and indeed, this is desirable to eliminate noise. A frequency response of 0.1 Hz to 1 Hz can therefore be recommended. An important feature is the very slow sweep speed of the oscilloscope beam. A 30-minute sweep is required and unfortunately such a slow rate of travel is not achievable on standard oscilloscopes. A suitable plug-in unit may be made in the local workshop, but if this is not possible then the idea of using an oscilloscope to record the electro-oculogram may have to be abandoned in favour of using a penwriting machine with a slow paper speed.

It is to be hoped that in future years the problem of obtaining and assembling several pieces of equipment will be solved by the existence of commercially available equipment. In fact combined 'packages' are already appearing on the market; these are suitable for routine clinical work but not perhaps so useful for research.

We have developed a system of automated electro-oculography which eliminates the need for a skilled assistant. A microprocessor is used to control the progress of the test and to calculate the result at the end. This result is read

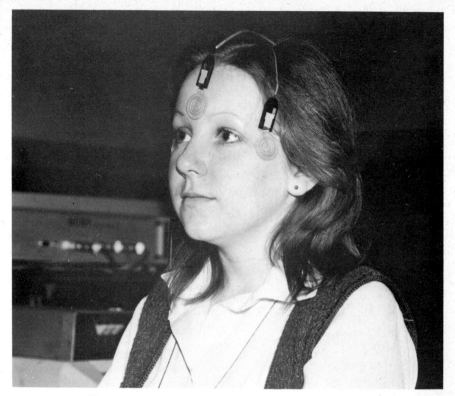

Figure 6.6. The electrodes in position for electro-oculography.

out on a teletype. The test can be carried out by a nurse and no special understanding of electronics is needed.

The visually evoked potential

Since this is still used largely for research purposes the type of stimulus that is chosen must depend on the particular research project that is envisaged. It is likely that some form of patterned stimulus will be required. The simplest way of producing a patterned stimulus is to illuminate a suitable pattern with a flashing light. This method has the disadvantage that the appearance and disappearance of the pattern is accompanied by luminance changes. Potentials produced by the change of luminance thus become confused with those produced by the pattern alone. Many different and ingenious methods have been devised to produce this type of stimulus. They have involved the use of twin projectors, rotating mirrors and polaroid discs. A detailed account of the types of stimuli used for producing a visually evoked response is given by Regan (1972).

The electrodes can be any of the standard types used for electro-encephalography, and the placement of the electrodes depends on the type of work involved. Signals from the scalp are fed into an isolated amplifier which must have a gain of approximately 50 000. The enlarged and repeated signals must then be processed by some form of averaging device. It is usual to examine the response of the scalp potentials for 500 msec after each flash. The responses from 100 flashes are absorbed by the averager and the averaged result is read out at the end of the test. A number of different averaging devices are available. For research purposes a small Nicolet computer can perform this function as well as many others and provides the most versatile answer to the problem. For routine clinical work, instruments are now produced commercially which have been designed solely for ophthalmic electrodiagnosis. That produced by Medelek is popular at present in this country.

In the next section the approximate cost of these instruments will be considered, but when costing a clinic of this sort it is important to remember the numerous other items such as chairs, shelves, a coatrack, etc. Not least of these is the provision of an effective lock on the door.

The Cost of the Clinic in the U.K.

Clearly, it is not possible to attempt any sort of accurate costing here, but the equipment for performing electroretinography and electro-oculography could cost about £5000 in the U.K. If visually evoked responses are also to be examined a further £15 000 or £20 000 may be required. Added to this are the cost of fixtures and fittings as well as running costs.

Running the Clinic

The flow of patients through an electrodiagnostic clinic must be carefully controlled. In the first instance it is important that one's colleagues are fully aware of the types of eye disease that can be most profitably examined by these techniques. If one is not careful the clinic time may be spent examining patients with retinitis pigmentosa. This may allow a fascinating and useful study of the condition, but it may interfere with the examination of other conditions. It may be considered useful to expand the function of the clinic to include detailed testing of colour vision and perhaps more important, the objective assessment of dark adaptation. It is advisable to keep separate notes for each patient and to file these in the clinic itself. It is also strongly advisable to organise an indexing system both diagnostic and numerical before the first patient arrives. This will circumvent much hard work at a later date.

After each patient has been examined the results can be typed on to a preprinted report sheet, or directly into the notes. An assistant is essential in the form of a nurse or technician, or preferably both, and this assistant should be shown how to set out the contact lenses and skin electrodes and other items needed for fitting the electrodes. A competent technician can be trained in about three months but it is probably preferable for the fitting of contact lenses to be done by medical staff in view of the risk of producing corneal abrasions. This decision may depend on the proved manual dexterity of the technician.

Once the clinic has been established, the running costs involve the purchase of Polaroid film and skin electrodes as well as the upkeep of equipment and contact lenses. They may also need to include a technician's salary.

REFERENCES

Krakau, C. & Öhman, R. (1975) Slit lamp ERG. *Acta Ophthalmologica (København)*, **125**, 9.
Regan, D. (1972) *Evoked Potentials in Psychology, Sensory Physiology and Clinical Medicine.* pp. 205–213. London: Chapman and Hall.

CHAPTER SEVEN

Recording a Normal Response

In this chapter the normal electrical changes induced by light in both the eye and brain will be considered in relation to the recording techniques used in clinical practice.

Newcomers to the electrodiagnostic scene may be confused by the apparent variation between the types of response obtained in different centres. At the early meetings of the International Society of Clinical Electroretinography* it was agreed that standardisation of the technique was very important. However, there are disadvantages in rigid standardisation of a new and unproved method of investigation if it limits experimentation. The value of standardisation in an individual clinic is undisputed, however, and it is only by the painstaking examination of enormous numbers of cases using an identical technique in each case that we have reached our present state of knowledge. At the present time many different centres have adapted their own special technique and normal values differ from place to place. It is likely that this situation will persist until electroretinogram equipment is miniaturised and marketed as a single package and until the full worth of each of the different methods of stimulation has been realised.

The human retina shows an electrical response to a flash of light which will vary according to the intensity, duration and colour of the light and the recorded response may also be modified by filters in the amplification system or by altering the sweep speed of the oscilloscope. If the eye is exposed to a prolonged light stimulus then the electrical response shows changes which occur over several minutes or longer. Unfortunately it is not possible to measure the immediate changes which occur within the first second with the same type of equipment that measures the long-term changes which occur over several minutes. The test which we employ for measuring the rapid part of the response is called the electroretinogram and the test for measuring the slow part of the response is called the electro-oculogram. Clearly it is a disadvantage to use two different pieces of equipment to measure different parts of the

* Now called the International Society for Clinical Electrophysiology of Vision (ISCEV).

same response, but so far there does not seem to be any satisfactory answer to this problem. The difficulty lies in the fact that the base line will not remain steady for more than a fraction of a second due to the slightest movements of the patient. The electroretinogram can be recorded during these brief moments when the base line is steady, but electro-oculography must be used to detect the slower changes, this being in reality a trick to eliminate the effect of base line variation.

If advances in medical electronics enabled us to record the total response with a single piece of equipment the trace would resemble that shown in Figure 7.1. Note that this is an idealised drawing of the response to a prolonged light stimulus. In the following pages we shall consider first of all the means of recording the response over the first 200 msec (the electroretinogram), and secondly the means of recording the slow changes which occur over half an hour (the electro-oculogram). Following this, the means of recording the equivalent electrical changes over the scalp will be considered. Although the classical electroretinogram is recorded as the response to a single flash of light, certain components of the response can only be seen if a special type of stimulus is used. For example, special methods must be employed to measure flicker fusion or to examine the electroretinogram from localised areas of the retina. The technique of averaging is also useful when applied to the electroretinogram, particularly when examining the oscillatory potential. Finally, we must not forget that an 'off effect' can be recorded in the human and this may have some clinical value in the future.

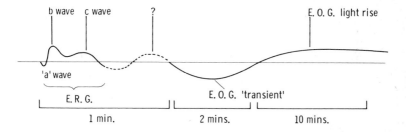

Figure 7.1. Diagram to illustrate the effect of a prolonged light stimulus on the corneo-retinal potential. The electroretinogram and electro-oculogram are represented on the same trace, although they cannot be recorded in this manner in the clinic.

The 'c' wave of the electroretinogram is not usually well shown by the standard methods of clinical electroretinography. It requires a prolonged flash to elicit it and it is a little too slow to be easily recorded, and yet it occurs too early to be seen on the electro-oculogram. In fact there is a 'no man's land' where our knowledge of the response in the human is lacking and this occurs between the end of the first half minute and the beginning of the second minute. An attempt to explore this area using an electro-oculographic technique is illustrated in Figure 7.2. This part of the trace has recently been carefully elucidated by Nilsson & Skoog (1975).

We are now in a position to consider how the normal response is recorded and what factors can cause variations in the response in a normal subject.

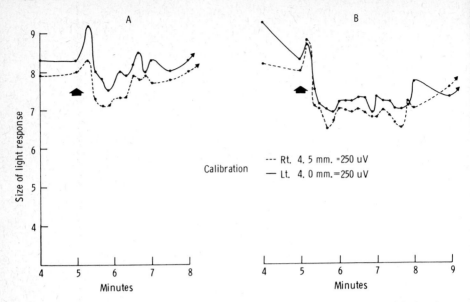

Figure 7.2. The electro-oculogram was recorded continuously from the point at which the stimulus light was switched on. Readings during the first few seconds are not accurate due to photophobia. However, in this series of experiments the brief negative transient prior to the light rise is well shown and this appears to be preceded by a positive wave. Vertical axis: millimetres of penwriter deflection; A: reduced light intensity; B: maximum intensity.

THE NORMAL ELECTRORETINOGRAM

Recording Techniques in Different Clinics

Although many different techniques are used throughout the world, it is fitting to begin by describing the method used by Karpe and co-workers in 1946. Like many other people, they found that to carry out the investigation after total dark adaptation was very time consuming for normal clinical practice. If the patient had been exposed to strong light prior to testing, dark adaptation for 30 minutes was carried out before the standardised part of dark adaptation was started in the electroretinogram recording room. After entering the recording room which had an illumination of 3 to 6 lux the subject was asked to lie on the examination couch and the pupil was dilated with Mydriacyl drops and the cornea anaesthetised with Ophthaine. A period of 20 minutes of semi-darkness (3 to 6 lux) was followed by five minutes in complete darkness and during this time the skin electrodes and the contact lens were placed in position. Using this technique the 'b' wave reaches a steady potential after three minutes total dark adaptation and retains it for about 30 minutes. The light that they used was an electric bulb fed via a condenser which gave a flash lasting 0.15 sec. Changes in the intensity of the light from 20 lux to 80 and 100 lux could be achieved by changing the distance between the bulb and the eye. A weak red fixation light was positioned immediately adjacent to the stimulus light. This type of stimulus gave a maximum 'b' wave response with the 20 lux stimulus in normal subjects and this could be confirmed by showing a reduction in the size of the 'b' wave with brighter flashes.

The time constant of the amplifier was 1.5 sec to 2.0 sec and recordings were made with a direct writing ink jet recorder (Mingograf 24B). Calibration of the response was achieved by passing a constant voltage of 0.5 mV through the amplifier and recorder. Records were taken from both eyes simultaneously. The 'b' wave value was taken from the mean of four readings and measured from the base line to the peak of the curve (Peterson, 1968).

A great number of variations on this technique exist; the period of dark adaptation varies from clinic to clinic and some centres favour the use of gas discharge tubes as a stimulus light. The penwriters and ink jet recorders are being replaced by the oscilloscope, a record being made by photographing the face of the oscilloscope using Polaroid film.

The technique used in our own clinic for routine purposes is designed to give as much information in as short a time as possible. We have dispensed with mydriasis and dark adaptation altogether. The patient enters the recording room directly and sits in a modified dental chair. After the skin electrodes have been placed on the cheek and forehead a drop of Ophthaine is instilled into each eye and the contact lenses are inserted. The contact lens and the types of skin electrode have been already described in the previous chapter. Once the contact lenses are in position and a good base line has been achieved, the stimulus flash is positioned and the result of a single flash is recorded. If the response is unsatisfactory the procedure is repeated after five minutes. The contact lenses and electrodes are then removed and the patient is allowed to leave. Because the test is so rapid and the wearing time of the contact lens is short, there is no residual discomfort and the patient is not inconvenienced by mydriasis. Our stimulus is an electronic flash lamp which gives a large response under light-adapted conditions. Precautions are taken to eliminate electrical and photoelectric artefacts from the beginning of the trace and this enables the early receptor potential to be recorded together with the 'a' wave, 'b' wave, and oscillatory wavelets.

In most clinics the standardised technique is supplemented by a method for measuring the response to flicker and also for measuring the response to different coloured stimuli. More sophisticated techniques are also used to elicit averaged electroretinogram responses and to detect the foveal electroretinogram and these will now be described.

The Averaged Electroretinogram

This method has the great advantage of eliminating much of the unwanted background 'noise' from the response and its use has been described by several authors (Jacobson, Stephens and Suzuki, 1962; Tassy, 1966; Stangos et al, 1970). Stangos et al in Geneva have used the following technique.

The corneal electrode led to an AC preamplifier (Tektronix type 122), the voltage gain being 100 times the input. The preamplifier was connected to a digital computer of average transients (Biomac 1000 of Data Laboratories), and also to a dual beam oscilloscope fitted with a Polaroid camera. A Grass PS2 photostimulator was used at two intensities, one being approximately 16 times the other. The examination was carried out as follows:

1. The pupils were dilated and the subject was light adapted for three minutes.

2. An average of 64 responses to the weaker flash was made at a frequency of one cycle/second.
3. An average of 64 responses to the higher intensity was made at the same frequency.
4. After light adapting for a further three minutes the average of 64 responses to a red stimulus was made. This technique shows up the oscillatory potential particularly well, as can be seen from Figure 7.3.

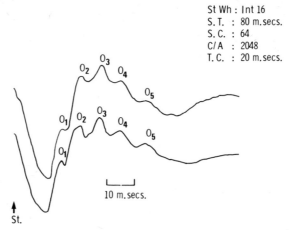

St Wh : Int 16
S. T. : 80 m.secs.
S. C. : 64
C/A : 2048
T. C. : 20 m.secs.

10 m.secs.

St.

Figure 7.3. An averaged electroretinogram in a normal subject. (St.Wh.Int.16: White stimulus intensity 16; S.T.: sweep time; S.C.: sweep count; C/A: counts address ratio; T.C.: time constant). Reproduced from Stangos, Rey, Meyer & Thorens (1970) *VIIIth Symposium of ISCERG*, 279, Fig. 1, (Ed.) A. Wirth. Pisa: Pacini, with permission.

The Foveal Electroretinogram

A technique for recording the foveal electroretinogram was described in 1966 (Arden and Bankes, 1966), and there is no doubt that this method can detect macular degeneration. However, its value in the presence of opaque media has yet to be proved. A standard contact lens was used and the stimulus was a back-illuminated diffuser 1.5 cm in diameter at 43 cm from the eye and subtending a visual angle of 2°. The front face of the diffuser was covered by a large piece of white card illuminated by a blue/green light. The stimulus flashes (150/min) were provided by a xenon stroboscope covered by a red filter. When the stimulus fell on the blind spot and there was no blue/green background, a diffuse electroretinogram could be obtained. The background intensity was then increased till the diffuse response disappeared. At this point the stimulus was shifted to the fovea and well-marked 'a' and 'b' waves could be recorded. The responses were much smaller if the stimulus colour was changed to green or blue. The size of the foveal response was about 10 μV; 150 responses were averaged to detect this, using a Mnemotron CAT.

Here, then, are a few examples of the different techniques which are practised in different clinics. The methods used in several other well-known electrodiagnostic clinics have been omitted to avoid repetition; the main point to note is that the normal values quoted by different clinics vary considerably and this is largely due to differences in intensity of the stimulus flash and to the varying periods of dark adaptation. This leads us to consider in more detail the numerous factors whicn can influence the normal response.

The Factors Influencing the Normal Electroretinogram

These may be summarised as follows:

1. Physiological variations:
   State of dark adaptation
   Pupil size
   Diurnal rhythm
   Refractive error
   Age and sex

2. Variations due to type or adjustment of equipment:
   Amplifier, setting of gain and time constant
   Type of recorder
   Electrode position
   Stimulus colour, duration and intensity

3. Variations in response due to artefacts:
   Blinking
   Tears
   Bubbles in contact lens
   Eye movements
   Photoelectric and electrical artefacts

Physiological Variations

The effect of dark adaptation

That the normal electroretinogram shows both photopic and scotopic characteristics became evident after Motokawa and Mita showed that the 'b' wave was in fact split into two. Thus the 'b' wave was shown to consist of a pointed wave (the 'x' wave), followed by a rounded wave which was the 'b' wave proper (Motokawi and Mita, 1942). Shortly after this Adrian showed that these two parts of the 'b' wave reflected rod and cone activity respectively. Armington and co-workers showed a similar splitting of the 'a' wave (Adrian, 1945; Armington, Johnson and Riggs, 1952). It has been shown that the earlier of the split components of both 'a' wave and 'b' wave predominate under light-adapted conditions, whereas the later components predominate under dark-adapted conditions. The effect becomes more evident if a red filter is used for the light-adapted response and a blue-filter is used for the dark-adapted response (Figure 7.4). However, although it is relatively easy to demonstrate clinically that the 'b' wave changes shape during dark adaptation and the later of its double peaks gradually increases in size (Figure 7.5), the changes in the 'a' wave are less clear and some still dispute that the 'a' wave has photopic and scotopic components.

As a general rule we can say that during dark adaptation the 'b' wave increases in size under constant stimulus conditions and that this increase in amplitude is accompanied by a change in shape.

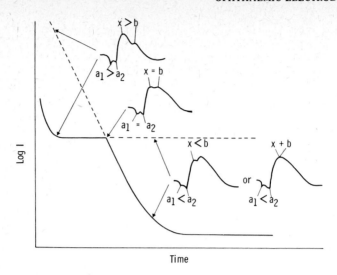

Figure 7.4. The evolution of separate components of the 'a' wave and the 'b' wave during the course of dark adaptation (Auerbach and Burian, 1955).

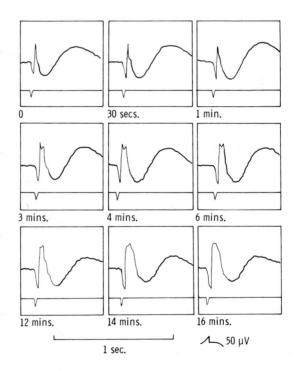

Figure 7.5. The recording of successive electroretinograms during dark adaptation showing the transition from the sharp photopic 'b' to the more rounded scotopic form. Reproduced from Duke-Elder (1962) *A System of Ophthalmology*, 7, 429. London: Henry Kimpton, with permission.

The effect of pupil size

It will be seen later in this chapter that the size of the 'b' wave is proportional to the square root of the stimulus intensity for weak flashes and to the log of the intensity, up to a certain limit, for stronger flashes. It is perhaps not surprising that these results can be modified by altering the size of the pupil. When the size of the pupil is fixed by mydriasis the 'b' wave increases in size with increasing intensity of stimulus until it reaches a maximum value. It has been shown that this maximum value is reached at higher stimulus intensity levels when the pupils are not dilated (Figure 7.6). Furthermore, the flicker fusion frequency varies with the size of the pupil. Different curves are obtained in the same subject depending on whether the pupil is dilated or constricted (Figure 7.7) (Karpe and Wulfing, 1961).

If we are only concerned with measuring the maximal size of the 'b' wave the size of the pupil is not important even though a slightly higher intensity stimulus may be needed to elicit it when the pupil is small. The pupil size can also influence the size of the 'a' wave and also the duration of the 'a' and 'b' waves, and for this reason in most clinics the pupils are dilated as part of the test. However, when high intensity flashes are used the electrical response occurs before the undilated pupil has time to react, and if the test is carried out in the dark the error introduced by pupil size is not very great. It must be remembered that mydriasis can cause considerable inconvenience to the patient and extra loss of time from work.

Diurnal rhythm and the electroretinogram

Although one might expect to find a diurnal variation in the electroretinogram since this is a common feature of biological responses, this has not so far been well shown in man. It is well known that the electroretinogram can

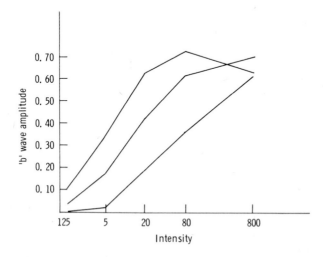

Figure 7.6. 'b' wave amplitudes plotted against stimulus intensity for different pupil sizes. When the pupil size is larger than 5 mm the 'b' wave reaches its maximal value at the same intensity irrespective of pupil size. Reproduced from Karpe & Wulfing (1961) *Acta Ophthalmologica,* **70,** 53, with permission.

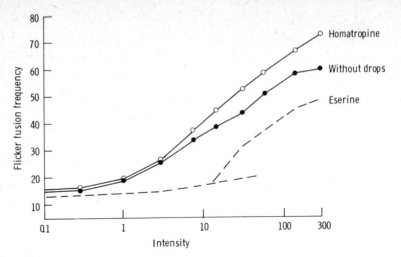

Figure 7.7. The relationship of the flicker fusion frequency (FFF) to pupil size. Reproduced from
Karpe & Wulfing (1961) *Acta Ophthalmologica*, **70**, with permission.

vary considerably in amplitude from day to day and month to month in a
given individual, and Figure 7.8 shows an example of this. In view of the
possibility of variations occurring in relation to the time of day it is advisable
to limit the testing of subjects for a normal series to the same time each day.

The investigation of the amplitude of the components of the electroretinogram at different times of day is not easy because it necessarily entails wearing
the contact lens electrode for prolonged periods and at many different times
of day. In an investigation of two subjects it was found that whereas in one

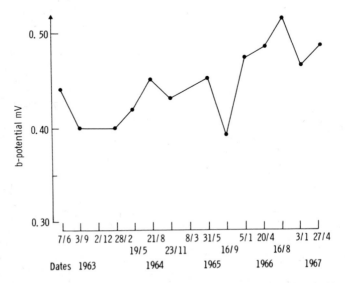

Figure 7.8 The 'b' potential recorded in the same patient on different occasions. Reproduced
from Peterson (1968) *Acta Ophthalmologica*, **99**, with permission.

case the electroretinogram recorded in the morning was smaller than that recorded in the afternoon, in the other case the findings were reversed (Ronchi and Ercoles, 1968). The variability of the electroretinogram and the factors which influence it from day to day and month to month clearly require more study.

The effect of refractive error on the response

Peterson reported on the relationship of the 'b' wave amplitude to refractive error in a series of 1136 normal eyes. These were divided into three groups. The first comprised persons with a refraction ranging from +2.0 to −1.0 D. This group was regarded as the normal group since the frequency peak of the refractive error lay at +0.5 D. The second group consisted of all the hypermetropes with an error of more than +2.25 D and the third group was composed of the myopes with a refractive error greater than −1.0 D. After allowing for age, it was shown that both myopic and hypermetropic women had a lower 'b' potential than those with normal refraction. The myopes differed more (−0.075 mV) than the hypermetropes (−0.050 mV). In males, however, although the myopes showed a lower 'b' potential than normal, the hypermetropes had a slightly higher response than normal. Probably the numbers in these groups are not large enough to allow firm conclusions to be drawn from these figures, but the lower response in myopes is well accepted and will be discussed further in the chapter on inherited disease.

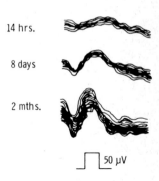

14 hrs.

8 days

2 mths.

⌐⌐ 50 µV

Figure 7.9. The response to a flash of 700 lux in the early months. Reproduced from Zetterström (1970) *The Electroretinogram of the Newborn Infant. VIIIth Symposium of ISCERG*, (Ed.) A. Wirth. Pisa: Pacini, with permission.

The effect of age and sex on the response

Earlier reports of the electroretinogram in newborn infants failed to find any response, but stronger stimuli can elicit a response within hours after birth. The electroretinogram probably reaches its adult value at the age of two years and in adult life it declines slightly with age, being slightly larger in women than in men. Using Karpe's technique, Zetterström showed that no electroretinogram could be recorded within the first few hours after birth and after a few days a small positive potential could be detected with a latent period of 0.06 sec (0.04 sec in an adult). At three months the amplitude of the 'b' wave was 0·1 to 0·2 mV. When a stronger stimulus was used a slow 'a' wave as well as a 'b' wave was visible 14 hours after birth (Zetterström, 1970) (Figure 7.9). Using a specially constructed stimulus flash Algvere and Zetterström have demonstrated the presence of the oscillatory potential in the newborn (Algvere and Zetterström, 1967).

The slow decline in the size of the 'b' potential with age has been well documented (Karpe, Rickenbach and Thomasson, 1950). In a series of 79 men and 52 women aged 19 to 50 years, the 'b' potential was significantly higher in women than in men (Vainio-Mattila, 1951). This has been confirmed in Peterson's series and it has been suggested that this difference is related to the shorter length of the eyeball in women. In 1950 Karpe gave the normal value for the 'b' wave amplitude as 0·30 mV in males and 0·34 mV in females. After the age of 60 years normal values were given as follows: 60 to 64 years—0·31 mV; 65 to 69 years—0·25 mV; 70 to 74 years—0·23 mV (Karpe, Rickenbach and Thomasson, 1950).

Variations due to Type or Adjustment of Equipment

Gain setting and time constant of the amplifier
Obviously any adjustment of the gain setting of the amplifier will alter the size of the trace and this setting must not be altered without recalibrating the response with a known signal. In practice the gain may have to be altered in order to allow a large signal to fit on the recording paper or film, or to enable the easier measurement of a very small signal. The significance of the time constant of the amplifier has been explained in the first chapter. When a fast time constant is used the equipment does not detect slow changes in potential. Time constants of 0·5 sec to 1·0 sec are commonly used in clinical practice and this may cause some apparent shortening of the 'b' wave. The shape of the response may also be markedly altered by adjusting the sweep speed of the oscilloscope or the paper speed of a penwriter. A faster sweep speed is usually employed for demonstrating the oscillatory wavelets and in such traces the waveform appears longer and more drawn out compared with the electroretinogram which is produced using Karpe's technique.

Type of recorder
Because of the inertia of the moving arm, pen recorders are not suitable for recording the more rapid components, such as the early receptor potential and the oscillatory wavelets. Pen recorders have the advantage of being able to display repeated responses on the same sheet, whereas the face of an oscilloscope can only accommodate single responses. However, the response from the oscilloscope is a more accurate one. When a Polaroid camera is used to photograph the face of the oscilloscope a further recording error may be introduced by the camera; some degree of barrel distortion may be present and the trace may be magnified on the film. Such errors can of course be taken into account and the measuring grid on the oscilloscope should be photographed with the trace.

Electrode position
It is fortunate that the type of contact lens electrode does not have much influence on the electroretinogram. The results of comparing several different types of commonly used lenses have been studied and the difference in the responses obtained was not significant (Sundmark, 1961). When recordings are made from different parts of the cornea the 'b' potential is found to be maximal and constant in size, but it decreases rapidly when the electrode is

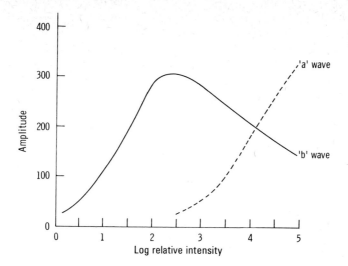

Figure 7.10. The relationship between stimulus intensity and 'a' and 'b' wave amplitudes. The positive 'a' wave and negative 'b' wave have been represented on the same side of the abscissa for simplicity. Reproduced from Peregrin & Sverak (1968) *Physiologia Bohemslovaca*, **17**, 338, Figure 2, with acknowledgement.

moved from the limbus posteriorly (Sundmark, 1959). The position of the cheek electrodes can alter the size of the response and this should be kept as constant as possible although variations in the conformity of the face may sometimes make this difficult.

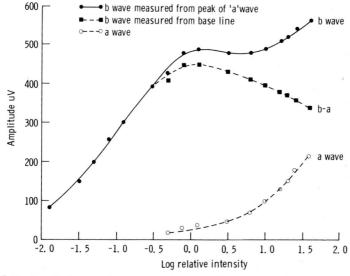

Figure 7.11. Amplitude intensity curves to show the effect of measuring the 'b' wave from the peak of the 'a' wave or from the base line. 'a' wave amplitudes are represented on the same side of the abscissa for simplicity. Reproduced from Burian & Pearlman (1964) *American Journal of Ophthalmology*, **58**, 212, Figure 1, with permission of authors and editor.

The nature of the stimulus

If the intensity of the stimulus is gradually increased under dark-adapted conditions, the amplitude of the 'b' wave also increases and eventually the rate of increase falls off until a maximum value is reached (between 400 μV and 500 μV). Beyond this point the amplitude of the 'b' wave diminishes with increase in intensity of the stimulus. This only applies if the 'b' wave is measured in the conventional manner from the base line to the peak. In some series the 'b' wave has been measured from the peak of the 'a' wave to the peak of the 'b' wave. Since the amplitude of the 'a' wave continues to increase with extra stimulus strength, it is important that the method of measurement of the 'b' wave is clearly defined (Figure 7.10), (Peregrin and Sverak, 1968; Burian and Pearlman, 1964). Because the electroretinogram is the sum of several different waveforms, the interpretation of these changes with intensity is not easy. For example, if the 'b' wave is measured from the peak of the 'a' wave to the peak of the 'b' wave, a graph showing the relationship between intensity of stimulus and amplitude has a different shape; although the curve levels off at higher intensities, it continues to rise again beyond this (Figure 7.11). The point at which the curve begins to rise again has been likened to the rod/cone break in the diphasic dark-adaptation curve (Burian and Pearlman, 1964).

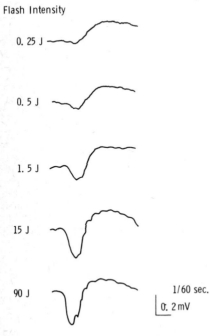

Flash Intensity

0. 25 J

0. 5 J

1. 5 J

15 J

90 J

1/60 sec.

0. 2 mV

Figure 7.12. The effect of increasing the stimulus intensity to higher levels on the response. Reproduced from Yonemura et al (1961) *Acta Ophthalmologica*, **70**, 118, Figure 4, with permission.

When the intensity of the stimulus flash is increased beyond the level which gives a maximum value for the 'b' wave, further changes are seen in the shape of the waveform. At these higher levels of intensity the oscillatory wavelets become visible (Figure 7.12). The increasing negativity of the response with the 'b' wave being pulled towards the base line is evident in the figure. As the intensity is increased still further, the early receptor potential begins to appear before the 'a' wave (see Figure 2.2, Chapter 2).

At this point we must consider the relationship between the splitting of the 'b' wave which is seen using coloured filters at lower intensities and the oscillatory potential which is seen at higher intensities. One way of looking at this is to regard the wavelets as a quite separate response superimposed on a smooth 'a' and 'b' wave. The wavelets have an almost fixed latency over a wide range of flash intensities whereas the latency of the 'a' and 'b' waves decreases as the intensity increases. The result of this is that the wavelets appear to move backwards and forwards along the trace for different light intensities. Thus at very high intensities they lie high up on the 'b' wave but at lower intensities they encroach on the 'a' wave. The wavelets are not well seen with dimmer flashes so that only one 'hump' may be visible, this being the 'x' wave. Figure 7.13 shows the traces obtained by a number of different workers with different flash intensities, and it indicates the present confusion of nomenclature. It is probably simplest to adopt the Japanese nomenclature and refer to the wavelets as 0_1, 0_2, etc. The electroretinogram literature is already confused by a multiplicity of capital letters.

The question of the nature and origin of the wavelets is considered in Chapter 2, but it is important to stress here that they appear to be quite separate from the 'a' and 'b' waves. They are selectively abolished in disease and show a constant latency at different flash intensities.

Less attention has been paid in the literature to the effect of the duration of the stimulus on the electroretinogram in the human. Bornschein and Gunkel found that with rise times from 25 to 100 msec, the 'a' wave amplitude was

HUMAN ERG

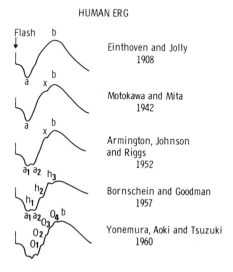

Figure 7.13. Examples of the different nomenclature which has been used to define the various humps on the 'a' and 'b' waves. Reproduced from Algvere (1968) *Acta Ophthalmologica*, **96**, 14, with permission.

reduced by half, while the amplitude of the 'b' wave remained constant. When the rise time was increased from 100 to 280 msec. the duration of the 'b' wave increased and the 'a' wave became unrecordable (Bornschein and Gunkel, 1956). In a similar experiment Burian showed that with increasing duration of square wave light flashes, the 'b' wave reached a maximum value when the stimulus duration was about 20 msec or longer. Very long stimuli gave a slightly smaller response. In clinical practice it is normal to use a brief flash of less than 20 msec, the idea being that the flash does not interfere with the waveform. However, if the 'off effect' or the 'c' wave are being studied a longer stimulus duration is required. When very intense flashes are used, they are usually produced by a xenon stroboscope or photoflash, and the duration of these flashes is usually very short, reaching a maximum in less than one millisecond.

It is disappointing that the electroretinogram as routinely recorded at present is a mass response and altering the area of retina stimulated does not have much effect. When it was shown that a good response could be obtained by stimulating the blind spot (Asher, 1951), it was evident that unavoidable scattering of light must occur. Francois and De Rouck carried out a study of the effect of changing the area of the light source, while maintaining constant illumination at the pupil. They showed that in photopic conditions a small area stimulus produced a considerably larger response than a diffuse stimulus. In scotopic conditions the 'a' wave became smaller with localised stimulation but the amplitude of the 'b' wave remained the same. Thus the 'b' wave seemed to be a more diffuse response when the subject was dark adapted (Francois and De Rouck, 1961).

Variation in the response due to artefacts

When weaker stimuli and a pen recorder are used, the effect of blinking becomes more important. In fact an isolated blink can sometimes look very like an electroretinogram. When the oscilloscope is used a blink is usually easily distinguished and the waveform of the electroretinogram with high intensity flashes is of course quite complex and characteristic. If a blink occurs coincidentally with the stimulus the trace is often lost from the face of the oscilloscope and the patient must be told to try and avoid blinking at the time the stimulus is applied. Tears can cause gross artefacts when they spill over the lid margins and if they come in contact with the cheek electrodes the response is usually lost altogether. Another source of artefacts is the presence of bubbles in the contact lens, and it is important to check for this if a satisfactory base line cannot be obtained. Eye movements and jaw clenching can also cause similar problems, but these can usually be easily avoided by warning the patient.

When the early receptor potential is being recorded, two further artefacts become important. The first is the photoelectric artefact. This can be eliminated by choosing a suitable material for the contact lens electrode such as stainless steel rather than silver, and by screening the contact lens electrode and the skin electrodes from the light. The second is the electrical artefact produced by the stimulus flash. This can be eliminated by carefully screening all the equipment and by making sure that the flash is not too close to the electrodes. Since a high intensity flash is needed this last condition can best be met by using some form of light guide.

Other causes of variation in the response

In spite of the fact that the known causes of variation in the response can be largely controlled there is still a considerable variation in the response between individuals. There are probably still many unknown factors which could account for this and their elucidation provides enormous scope for future research.

Types of Normal Electroretinogram

Photopic and scotopic electroretinograms

The electrical response of the dark-adapted retina to a white flash reflects both rod and cone activity, but in the clinic it is often useful to be able to separate these. This may be achieved in the following way:

1. If a flickering light is used with a frequency of 30 cycles per second, then a pure cone response results because the rod system cannot respond at this rate.
2. A pure cone electroretinogram can also be produced if the stimulus is superimposed on a steady background illumination. The background illumination serves to saturate the rods so that they cannot respond to brief flashes.
3. A rod response can be produced by stimulating the dark-adapted retina with a dim blue light which is below the cone threshold.
4. If a red light of suitable intensity is used a double peak can be seen on the 'b' wave and it has been widely accepted that the first peak represents a cone response and the second peak represents a rod response.

The response to an intense flash

It has already been mentioned that in our own clinic we use an intense flash as stimulus. Our light source is a photoflash of 45 J, the power pack being charged from the mains. Unfortunately there is not a satisfactory way of calibrating this rather rapid flash which peaks at 250 μsec. It is therefore difficult to compare the results obtained by this technique with those of Karpe using a flash of 200 lux. Certain special features appear in the response when this type of stimulus is used. Firstly the early receptor potential can be seen immediately prior to the 'a' wave; the 'a' wave is abnormally large and the 'b' wave is extremely small. However, if the 'b' wave is measured from the peak of the 'a' wave to the peak of the 'b' wave, then the size of this wave is not greatly different from the 'b' wave obtained by Karpe's technique. A further feature of this type of response is the prominence of the oscillatory potential and finally there is a pronounced refractory period after each response. If the stimulus is repeated half a minute after the first one, then the resulting response is half the size of the first. A repeat flash within two or three seconds of the first one produces no response whatsoever. Subjectively, a flash of this sort produces a dense after-image which changes colour over a period of half to three quarters of a minute and then disappears. In a series of 40 normal eyes the results were as follows:

Early Receptor Potential: Mean amplitude   222·7 µV
                                Standard deviation 103·6

'a' wave amplitude: Mean amplitude   326·1 µV
                                Standard deviation 101·4

'b'+'a' amplitude: Mean amplitude   332·9 µV
i.e. peak to peak   Standard deviation   93·4

Figure 7.14 shows a typical normal response from a photoflash.

Flicker

It has been shown that one method of obtaining a photopic electroretinogram is to present the eye with a rapid series of flashes. if a stimulus flash is repeated every few seconds using a weak stimulus, then the second response resembles

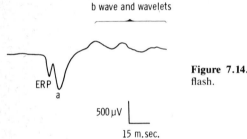

Figure 7.14. Typical normal response from a photoflash.

a normal electroretinogram. If the flash rate is increased to two per second then the second response and successive responses have a photopic character and are reduced in amplitude. As the frequency is increased the amplitude of 'a' and 'b' waves approach one another and beyond a certain frequency the trace becomes sinusoidal and finally it flattens off altogether when the critical fusion frequency is reached. The critical fusion frequency varies with the intensity of the stimulus. If a graph is made of intensity values against critical fusion frequency, then the resulting curve has a kink in it at about 20 per second. This kink corresponds with the rod/cone break in the dark adaptation curve and it suggests that the rods are not responding above the level of about 20 per second. With high intensities a fusion frequency of 70 per second can be reached (Dodt and Wadensten, 1954).

The 'off effect'

As a rule the clinical electroretinogram is recorded using a brief stimulus flash whose duration is limited to less than 20 msec. However, if a more prolonged stimulus is used then a change in electrical activity is evident when the stimulus is discontinued. In animal experiments this has been termed the 'off effect' or 'd' wave, but it has never been exploited clinically. It is known that the human 'off effect' is a negative going wave with a weak stimulus but becomes a positive wave as the stimulus is increased in intensity. The clinical applications of this have been limited, but it has been shown that the negative going wave elicited by a dim stimulus is absent in congenital stationary night blindness, but present in patients with rod monochromatopsia (Kawasaki, Tsuchida and Jacobson, 1971). It has also been shown that a series of wavelets may be found on the 'off effect' which bear a resemblance to the oscillatory potential (Tsuchida, Kawasaki and Jacobson, 1971). Nilsson has developed a DC registration technique which has allowed a more detailed study of the off-effect. After a very fast positive 'd' wave, a fast negative change occurs (the 'f' wave), a slower positive wave with a maximum at 0·9 to 1·5 sec. after 'off' (the 'g' wave), and a slow negative change with a maximum at 4 to 6 sec. (the 'h' wave). The 'h' wave seems to be the 'off' equivalent of the 'c' wave. (Skoog, Nilsson, and Welinder, 1978).

The averaged electroretinogram

The technique of averaging has been very helpful to the electroretinographer in that it enables very small signals to be detected and it has allowed us to see more detail on larger responses than would otherwise have been possible. In fact the work on the 'off effect' which is mentioned above made use of an averager. It is important to remember that averaging necessarily entails the measurement of a series of responses as opposed to isolated responses and often the light-adapting effect of the recurring stimulus must be taken into account. After the selected number of responses has been recorded in the memory of the averager the final result can be read out on the face of an oscilloscope. The resulting trace may sometimes be seen as a series of dots rather than a continuous line and the quality of the trace depends to some extent on the number of 'bits' in the memory store.

THE NORMAL ELECTRO-OCULOGRAM

Recording Techniques in Different Clinics

As has been explained, the principle of electro-oculography entails a method for measuring slow changes in the corneo-retinal potential by observing the fluctuating influence of the corneo-retinal potential during eye movements.

The technique of Francois, Verriest and De Rouck

Skin electrodes were placed on the temporal region lateral to the lateral canthi, and also on the side of the nose adjacent to the medial canthus. The indifferent electrode was placed occipitally. The active electrodes were made of silver and prior to their application the skin was wiped with ether. The subject was asked to make extreme lateral eye movements without blinking and as rapidly as possible. An inkwriter of a type used in electro-encephalography was employed with a time constant of 0·2 sec. A base line value of the electro-oculogram was first achieved by adapting the subject to a light of 10 lux for 10 minutes. The subject was then made to look into a bright light for five minutes; a Goldman-Weekers dark adaptometer was used for this purpose and after exposure the subject was placed in complete darkness for a further 15 or 20 minutes. The subject was asked to make eye movement at regular intervals during this total period and the excursions of the penwriter

were measured. As has been explained before, these excursions were related
to the corneo-retinal potential. Figure 7.15 shows the changes in the resting
potential which occur during the test in normal subjects. The following measurements were made:

1. The difference between the size of excursions on the penwriter after three
   minutes in the dark and the minimum excursions in the dark.
2. The value of the 'base line' after ten minutes adaptation to a light of 10
   lux.

This test was described by Francois, Verriest and De Rouck (1956). However, in 1962 more detailed investigations of the effect of light on the slow
changes in the corneo-retinal potential were made and a modification of this
test was developed by Arden and co-workers (Arden, Barrada and Kelsey,
1962). They discovered that if the eye is illuminated the corneo-retinal potential increases to a maximum and then begins to fall again, even though the
stimulus light is kept switched on. If the test is continued it can be seen that a
series of slow damped oscillations develop under constant illumination.

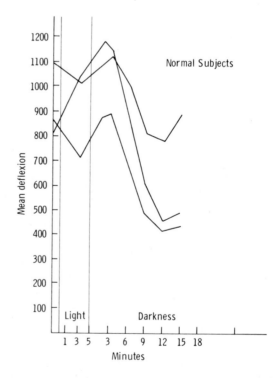

Figure 7.15. Serial measurement of the 'eye movement response' using the method of Francois et
al. Rise and fall of the curve indicates rise and fall of the corneo-retinal potential in light and
dark. Reproduced from Franceschetti, Francois & Babel (1963) *Les Heredo-dégénérescences
Choriorétiniennes.* Paris: Masson et Cie, with permission.

The technique of Arden, Barrada and Kelsey

Skin electrodes are placed in a similar manner to that of Francois, Verriest and De Rouck, and recordings are also made on a penwriter. The subject is asked to look to and fro between two fixation lights. Eye movements are carried out for a few seconds every minute, first of all for 12 minutes in the dark and then for about 10 minutes during exposure to a bank of strip lights. A ratio was made from the lowest value of the corneo-retinal potential in the dark and the maximum value in the light and this ratio has now become known as the Arden Index. Examples of a normal trace and the method of calculating the Arden Index are shown in Figure 7.16. Examination of a series of normal subjects has shown that the Arden Index can only be considered abnormal if it is below 185 per cent. In fact many patients with myopia and no other ocular pathology may show a value somewhat lower than this (Arden, Barrada and Kelsey, 1962). The histogram of this normal series showed that the frequency of the ratios was positively skewed, with the upper limit tailing off to levels approaching 400 per cent. The ratios of the two eyes were also closely correlated.

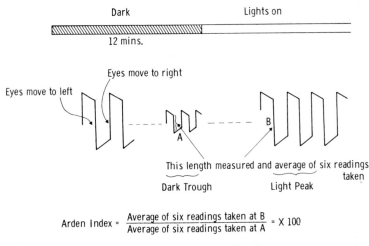

$$\text{Arden Index} = \frac{\text{Average of six readings taken at B}}{\text{Average of six readings taken at A}} = \text{X } 100$$

Figure 7.16. See text for explanation.

Variations of the normal electro-oculogram with time have been studied by Kelsey (1967). Eight subjects were tested weekly for at least ten weeks. The arithmetical mean of the ratios of the two eyes varied from 196 per cent to 304 per cent. Wide fluctuations of the Arden Index with time were apparent and this fluctuation appeared to be quite random. For example, in one subject the electro-oculogram varied between 250 per cent and 340 per cent over an 11-week period. Figure 7.17 shows the findings in these cases. All were female students aged between 18 and 25 years and the figure shows that no correlation between the electro-oculogram light ratio and ovulation could be seen.

Although the electro-oculogram has the advantage that it is not necessary to instil a contact lens, the test is rather lengthy and in its original form involved tedious calculations to obtain the Arden Index. When the test was first introduced each series of eye movements was represented as a series of

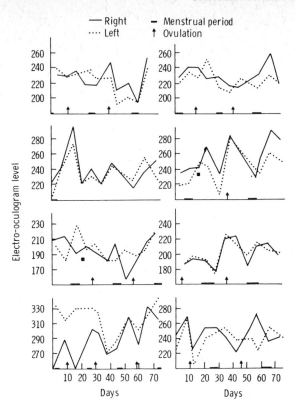

Figure 7.17. Variations in the electro-oculogram with time. Reproduced from Kelsey, J. H. (1967) *British Journal of Ophthalmology*, **51**, 47, Figure 1, with permission of author and editor.

square waves on the paper and six of these were separately measured and averaged. The averaged value of six excursions was thus obtained each minute and this value gradually decreased in the dark and then increased again when the lights were switched on. It was subsequently found that time could be saved if the paper speed of the penwriter was slowed down so that the pen excursions due to eye movements were compressed together. Using this method a value for the size of the excursions could be obtained almost at a glance and the saving on write-out paper was considerable. A more important development of the technique was achieved by Henkes and co-workers. They replaced the penwriter with an oscilloscope with a very slow time base. The light spot took half an hour to run across the face of the instrument. When the subject was asked to make eye movements these showed as a vertical bar on the screen which could be easily measured (Figure 7.18). The equipment was also modified to the extent that a selective amplifier was used; this was designed to record eye movements at a certain frequency only and eye movements at the correct speed were achieved by the alternate flashing of a pair of fixation lights. By this means irregularities in the trace could be considerably reduced. Instructions to the patient were also recorded on tape to simplify the technician's job (Henkes et al, 1968).

In our clinic we employ a development of Henke's method in which all the measurements and calculations are done electronically and the value of the Arden Index appears at the end of the test as a number printed on a teletype read-out together with a graph showing the light rise. The test in this form requires a minimum of technical skill from the operator. This device, which uses a microprocessor, is proving more satisfactory than our previous automated version of the electro-oculogram (Galloway and Barber, 1973).

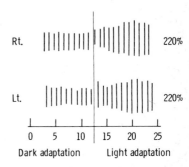

Figure 7.18. Electro-oculogram bar figures. The Arden Index is written at the right-hand side of the trace.

A method for recording the electro-oculogram in anaesthetised human subjects has been developed. Eye movements are achieved by means of low vacuum contact lenses attached to long shafts. This is an ingenious answer to the problem of the child who is not sufficiently co-operative, but sometimes an electroretinogram can be performed under these circumstances without the need for an anaesthetic (Henkes and Verduin, 1963).

RECORDING A NORMAL VISUALLY EVOKED POTENTIAL

The method of recording the visually evoked potential varies considerably from centre to centre. A major point of confusion arises from the fact that there is as yet no agreement as to which way up the trace should be recorded. In clinics which have previously been concerned largely with clinical electro-encephalography, the convention is to have negative upwards, and in clinics with a background of pure science or ocular electrophysiology the convention is to have positive upwards. To complete this Tower of Babel a wide range of types of stimulus and recording equipment are used. The present lack of clinical standardisation reflects a need for more research, but in spite of this some useful results are beginning to emerge concerning the nature of the normal response, and some of these will be considered here.

The following factors influence the normal VEP:

Stimulus

The VEP to a flash stimulus increases in amplitude with an increase in stimulus intensity, but a saturation point is reached. The latency is also reduced with an increase in intensity. Dark adaptation can be demonstrated with a VEP, as it can with the ERG, and a rod/cone break has been shown. A possibly useful clinical application of the VEP was realised when it became known that the response to a flash was relatively large, with a small centrally located stimulus. This appeared to reflect the wide area of macular representation on the occipital cortex. The VEP can therefore be used as a test of macular function (Rietveld, Tordoir and Duyff, 1965; Thompson and Harding, 1978).

Even though the response to an unstructured stimulus has been proved to be of some clinical value, pattern stimuli are now widely preferred, because the response to a pattern is much larger and bears a closer relationship to the act of seeing. Thus it has been shown that small patterns give a relatively large response when viewed by the macular area, whereas progressively larger patterns give a maximal response as the more peripheral parts of the retina are stimulated (Harter, 1970). It has already been mentioned in an earlier chapter that the frequency of the stimulus has a profound influence on the type of trace that can be obtained. Higher frequencies of stimulation, 10 or more Hz, make the test quicker and are probably more satisfactory to use from the technical point of view. On the other hand, low-frequency stimulation produces a more detailed response (the so-called transient response), and it is likely that this will hold more useful clinical information. A completely different approach from the stimulus point of view has been made by recording the trans-scleral VER. This is elicited by light delivered through an optical probe on the lower lid. The method has some promise when investigating retinal function in the presence of opaque media (Rubin and Dawson, 1978).

Age and sex differences in the response

During maturation the occipital VEP shows a rapid increase in amplitude of most components during early childhood, reaching a maximum in six- to eight-year-old children: at this age the VEP may be more than twice as large as that obtained in older age groups. After this peak there appears to be a decline in amplitude associated with increasing age until the thirteen to fourteen age group, when an abrupt increase is seen especially in the earlier components occurring in the first 200 milliseconds. The amplitude of the VEP seems to become stabilised at about the age of sixteen, showing a subsequent gradual reduction throughout life, and then declines rapidly in old age. The difference between male and female responses is not great, although female responses appear to be larger during adolescence and in adults, whereas male responses are larger in childhood. (Dustman et al, 1977).

Electrode position

Recording the VEP from a single electrode placed above the inion reveals only a small facet of the total response; for clinical purposes it is essential that an array of electrodes is used across the back of the scalp. The electrical changes from each electrode vary from millisecond to millisecond in a different manner at each electrode. This means that the response over a period of 500 milliseconds following the stimulus flickers across the scalp like light from moving water. Methods have now been worked out to represent this graphically or as spaciotemporal maps (Halliday et al, 1977). Again it must be remembered that these results depend on the type of stimulus being presented and may vary greatly depending on whether this is flashed pattern, pattern onset or pattern reversal.

Anatomical variations

The amplitude of the VEP differs markedly from subject to subject, and although not yet clearly shown, it is presumed that much of this variation is due to anatomical differences such as the thickness of the skull or the orientation of the occipital cortex in relation to the scalp. This is borne out by studies on identical twins, who showed very similar responses, and by the fact that in a given individual the response is very repeatable from day to day and hour to hour.

Other factors that may influence the response

Unfortunately, accurate recording of the VEP depends on subject co-operation and may be influenced by attention, fixation, and focusing. A malingerer could fool the machine by deliberately defocusing his eyes from the pattern or by fixing on a point elsewhere in the room. The problem of fixation in children can be overcome by presenting a television image in the centre of the screen to attract the child's attention. It is of course essential that the patient's correct spectacle prescription is worn at the time of the test.

In this chapter we have seen how normal electroretinograms, electro-oculograms and VEPs are recorded and how the technique is still being developed from year to year. Possibly our methods are still unacceptable for the clinician and the equipment and methods must be simplified further if their full value is to be realised. Apart from the complexity of the equipment, a further problem is the large variation of normal values, not only between individuals but also in a given individual. Perhaps in the future a better understanding of the cause of these variations will increase the accuracy and hence the clinical value of these tests.

REFERENCES

Adrian, E. D. (1945) The electric response of the human eye. *Journal of Physiology* (London), **104**, 84.

Algvere, P. (1968) Studies on the oscillatory potential of the clinical electroretinogram. *Acta Ophthalmologica* (Kobenhavn), **96**, 14.

Algvere, P. & Zetterström, B. (1967) Size and shape of the electroretinogram in newborn infants. *Acta Ophthalmologica* (Kobenhavn), **45**, 399–410.

Arden, G. B. & Bankes, J. L. K. (1966) Foveal electroretinogram as a clinical test. *British Journal of Ophthalmology*, **50**, 740.

Arden, G. B., Barrada, A. & Kelsey, J. H. (1962) New clinical test of retinal function based upon the standing potential of the eye. *British Journal of Ophthalmology*, **46**, 449–467.

Armington, J. C., Johnson, E. P. & Riggs, L. A. (1952) The scotopic 'a' wave in the electrical response of the human retina. *Journal of Physiology* (London), **118**, 289.

Asher, H. (1951) The electroretinogram of the blind spot. *Journal of Physiology* (London), **112**, 40.

Auerbach, E. & Burian, H. M. (1955) *American Journal of Ophthalmology* (Chicago), **40**, No. 5.

Bornschein, H. & Gunkel, R. D. (1956) The effect of rate of rise of photopic stimuli on the human electroretinogram. *American Journal of Ophthalmology*, **42**, 239–243.

Burian, H. M. & Pearlman, J. T. (1964) Evaluation of the 'b' wave of the human electroretinogram; its intensity, dependence and relation of the 'a' wave. *American Journal of Ophthalmology*. **58**, 210.

Dodt, E. & Wadensten, L. (1954) The use of flicker electroretinography in the human eye. *Acta Ophthalmologica* (Kobenhavn), **32**, 165–180.

Duke-Elder, Sir Stewart (1962) *A System of Ophthalmology*, **7**, 429. London: Henry Kimpton.

Dustman, R. E., Schenkenberg, T., Lewis, E. G. & Beck, E. C. (1977) *The Cerebral Evoked*

Potentials in Man: new developments. Ed. J. E. Desmedt. pp. 363–77. Oxford: Clarendon Press.

Franceschetti, A., Francois, J. & Babel, J. (1963) *Les Heredo-Dégénérescences Choriorétiniennes,* **1,** 226–306. Paris: Masson.

Francois, J. & De Rouck, A. (1961) A comparative study of the electroretinogram obtained by stimulation with diffuse light and with a small area stimulus. 1st ISCERG Symposium. *Acta Ophthalmologica* (Kobenhavn), **70,** 70–85.

Francois, J., Verriest, G. & De Rouck, A. (1956) Electro-oculography as a functional test in pathological conditions of the fundus. 1. First results. *British Journal of Ophthalmology,* **40,** 108–112.

Galloway, N. R. & Barber, C. (1973) Automated electro-oculography. *Transactions of the Ophthalmological Society of the United Kingdom,* **93,** 269–275.

Halliday, A. M., Barrett, G., Halliday, E. & Michael, W. F. (1977) The topography of the pattern evoked potential. In *Visual Evoked Potentials in Man: new developments* Ed. J. E. Desmedt. pp. 121–133. Oxford: Clarendon Press.

Harter, M. R. (1970) Evoked cortical responses to checkerboard patterns: effects of check size as a function of retinal eccentricity. *Vision Research* **10,** 1365–76.

Henkes, H. E., Denier, Van der Gon, J. J., Van Marle, G. W. & Schreinemachera, H. P. (1968) Electro-oculography: a semi-automatic recording procedure. *British Journal of Ophthalmology,* **52,** 122.

Henkes, H. E. & Verduin, P. C. (1963) Dysgenesis or abiotrophy? A differentiation with the help of the electroretinogram and electro-oculogram in Leber's congenital amaurosis. *Ophthalmologica* (Basel), **145,** 144–160.

Jacobson, J. J., Stephens, G. & Suzuki, T. (1962) Computer analysis of the electroretinogram. *Acta Ophthalmologica* (Kobenhavn), **40,** 313–319.

Karpe, G. (1945) The basis of clinical electroretinography. *Acta Ophthalmologica* (Kobenhavn), Suppl. **24,** 1.

Karpe, G., Rickenbach, K. & Thomasson, S. (1950) The clinical electroretinogram. (1) The normal electroretinogram above 50 years of age. *Acta Ophthalmologica* (Kobenhavn), **28,** 301–305.

Karpe, G. & Wulfing, B. (1961) Importance of pupil size in clinical electroretinogram. *Acta Ophthalmologica* (Kobenhavn), **70,** 53–54.

Kawasaki, K., Tsuchida, Y. & Jacobson, J. H. (1971) Positive and negative deflections in the off-response of the electroretinogram in man. *American Journal of Ophthalmology,* **72,** 367–375.

Kelsey, J. H. (1967) Variations in the normal electro-oculogram. *British Journal of Ophthalmology,* **51,** 44–49.

Motokawa, K. & Mita, T. (1942) Ueber eine einfachere Untersuchungsmethode und Eigenschaften der Aktionsströme der Netzhaut de Menschen. *Tohoku Journal of Experimental Medicine,* **42,** 114–133.

Nilsson, S. E. G. & Skoog, K. O. (1975) Covariation of the simultaneously recorded 'c' wave and the standing potential of the human eye. *Acta Ophthalmologica* (Kobenhavn), **53,** 721–730.

Peterson, H. (1968) The normal 'b' potential in the single-flash E.R.G. A computer technique study of the influence of age and sex. *Acta Ophthalmologica* (Kobenhavn), Suppl. **99.**

Rietveld, W. J., Tordoir, W. E. M. & Duyff, J. W. (1965) The contribution of fovea and parafovea to the visual evoked response. *Acta Physiologica et Pharmacologica Neerlandica,* **13,** 330–339.

Ronchi, L. & Ercoles, A. M. (1968) Circadian electroretinographic rhythms. *Atti della Fondazione e Contributi dell'Istituto Nazionale di Ottica* (Firenze), **23,** 92.

Rubin, M. L. & Dawson, W. W. (1978) The trans-scleral VER: Prediction of post-operative acuity. *Investigative Ophthalmology and Visual Science,* **17,** 71–74.

Skoog, K. O., Nilsson, S. E. G. & Welinder, E. (1978) Slow off-effects of the human DC registered ERG. *Documenta Ophthalmologica* (Proceedings Series), **15,** 114.

Stangos, H., Rey, P., Meyer, J. J. & Thorens, B. (1970) Average responses in normal human subjects and ophthalmological patients. *VIIth Symposium of ISCERG.* (Ed.) Wirth, Alberto. Pisa: Pacini.

Sundmark, E. (1959) The contact glass in human electroretinography. *Acta Ophthalmologica* (Kobenhavn), **52.**

Sundmark, E. (1961) Electroretinogram recordings with different types of contact glass. *Acta Ophthalmologica* (Kobenhavn), **70,** 62–68.

Tassy, A. F. (1966) *The Use of Averaging in Ophthalmologic Electrophysiology and Electro-diagnosis*. Medical Thesis, Marseille.

Thompson, C. R. S. & Harding, G. F. A. (1978) The visual evoked potential in patients with cateracts. *Documenta Ophthalmologica* (Proceedings Series), **15**, 193–201.

Tsuchida, Y., Kawasaki, K. & Jacobson, J. H. (1971) Rhythmic wavelets of the positive off-effect in the human electroretinogram. *American Journal of Ophthalmology*, **72**, 60–79.

Vainio-Mattila, B. (1951) The clinical electroretinogram: The difference between the electro-retinogram in men and women. *Acta Ophthalmologica* (Kobenhavn), **29**, 25–32.

Yonemura, D., Tsukudi, K. & Aoki, T. (1961) The clinical importance of oscillatory potentials in the human electroretinogram. *1st ISCERG Symposium*, **70**, 115. (Published 1962.)

Zetterström, B. (1970) The electroretinogram of the newborn infant. *VIIth ISCERG Symposium (Pisa)* pp. 1–9. (Ed.) Wirth, Alberto. Pisa: Pacini.

CHAPTER EIGHT

The Inherited Degenerations of the Retina

Under this heading 'Inherited degeneration of the retina', it is proposed to consider the electrical responses in a wide group of diseases, all of which have a hereditary tendency and many of which are progressive and may lead to blindness. A common feature is the presence of pigment in the retina which has migrated from the pigment epithelium. Many of these conditions are associated with night blindness at an early stage in the disease process.

It was in the investigation of this group of diseases some thirty years ago that the electroretinogram began to show some clinical value. From the turn of the century until that time the clinical applications had barely been investigated and indeed some research workers felt then that its use would always be restricted to the laboratory. However, the work of Karpe (1945), and that of very many others since then, has shown that pronounced changes occur in the electroretinogram at an early stage in the development of inherited retinal degenerations. This discovery led to the realisation that diffuse disease of the retina may cause alterations in the electroretinogram which are out of proportion to the ophthalmoscopic appearances, and in some instances the electroretinogram may be abnormal when the fundus appears normal to the ophthalmoscopist.

The hereditary nature of these conditions opened further pathways for research since it was possible to examine relatives of affected patients in an attempt to detect the disease at an early stage, and also to examine suspected carriers for latent defects of retinal function.

Unfortunately, at the present time there is no effective treatment for the progressive retinal degenerations and this necessarily limits the value of any diagnostic technique. However, we shall see later that the possibility of treatment is perhaps not as remote as one may think for some of these disorders.

CLASSIFICATION

I. *Progressive degenerations*
  a. Peripheral
     1. Retinitis pigmentosa
     2. Atypical forms of retinitis pigmentosa
     3. Retinitis punctata albescens
     4. Leber's amaurosis
  b. Central
     1. Central retinitis pigmentosa
     2. Progressive cone dystrophy
     3. Heredomacular dystrophies
  c. Associated with choroidal degeneration
     1. Choroideremia
     2. Gyrate atrophy
     3. Choroidal sclerosis
     4. Sorsby's pseudo-inflammatory dystrophy
     5. Myopic degeneration
     6. Angioid streaks
  d. Associated with vitreous degeneration
  e. Associated with systemic disease

II. *Related stationary conditions;*
  a. Associated with night blindness
     1. Congenital night blindness with normal fundi
     2. Fundus albipunctatus
     3. Fundus flavimaculatus
     4. Oguchi's disease
     5. Congenital fleck retina
  b. Without night blindness
     1. Congenital grouped pigmentation
     2. Sjögren's reticular dystrophy

In this classification the term 'tapeto-retinal degeneration' has been avoided although it is often applied to this group of diseases. It was originally used by Leber (Duke-Elder, 1967) who believed that the primary fault in these conditions lay in the pigment epithelium or 'tapetum nigrum'. Some confusion is added by using the expression 'tapetal reflex' when referring to the appearance seen in some cases of retinitis pigmentosa and in particular in the female carriers of sex-linked retinitis pigmentosa. It has been likened to the tapetal reflex seen in animals other than man where the normal presence of a tapetum gives this effect (Falls and Cotterman, 1948).

The overlap between these different conditions which may be seen in individual cases and the fact that many transitional forms may be seen in the same pedigree suggests a similar pathogenesis in all cases and this is perhaps borne out by the striking changes which are evident in the electroretinogram.

The results of performing electrodiagnostic procedures on patients suffering from these conditions will now be considered together with a brief description of the condition itself. For a detailed description of the clinical picture the reader is referred to more comprehensive textbooks on the subject (Franceschetti, Francois and Babel, 1963; Duke-Elder, 1967).

Peripheral Progressive Degenerations

Retinitis Pigmentosa

Retinitis pigmentosa was originally described by Donders in 1855, who noted the appearance of abnormal pigment in blind eyes shortly after the invention of the ophthalmoscope (Donders, 1855). Von Graefe three years later called attention to the hereditary nature of the condition (Von Graefe, 1858). Much of the detailed work on the inheritance was performed in this country after the turn of the century.

The disease is characterised by a degenerative process which begins in the outer layers of the retina and at first selectively involves the rods. Gradually all the layers of the retina become affected as well as the choriocapillaris accompanied by gliosis and pigment migration.

More recently much research interest has been centred on the relationship between retinitis pigmentosa and certain systemic disorders where there is a known inborn error of metabolism. These will be discussed later in this chapter.

Presenting features of retinitis pigmentosa

History. Many patients with this condition are unaware of the disorder until it is diagnosed during the course of a routine spectacle check. It is suprising that night blindness may be unnoticed by the patient until it is quite severe. Eventually the patient becomes aware of a constricted visual field, and this may progress to the extent that reading vision may be retained when he or she is blind for most other purposes.

Family history. The disease may be inherited as an autosomal recessive, autosomal dominant or X-linked recessive trait. There is wide agreement that the recessive form is by far the commonest, with the autosomal dominant being less frequent and the X-linked type being the rarest. The female carriers of this type commonly show a variety of fundus abnormalities and yet functional abnormalities are minimal. A number of patients who present with retinitis pigmentosa have no family history and these are sometimes termed sporadic cases; however, conclusions regarding inheritance with only one affected member of the family can only be speculative (Krill, 1972). As a general rule the severity of the disease and the rate of progress depend upon the mode of inheritance and the electroretinogram has been particularly valuable as an objective means of assessing this. The autosomal recessive form of the disease shows marked changes of retinal function at an early stage and the progress is usually rapid with a high incidence of ocular complications such as macular degeneration and complicated cataracts. The autosomal dominant type has relatively mild findings initially and a slowly progressive course. However, in some recessive cases the onset may be late and progress slow and these seem to form a separate rare group.

Fundus changes. The most striking fundus feature is the presence of scattered pigmentation in the equatorial region, the pigment being arranged in the pattern of 'bone spicules'. In places it may be distributed along the peripheral retinal veins. The retinal vessels become narrowed and in advanced cases may be so narrow in places that they are scarcely visible. The optic disc is atrophic and has a characteristic waxy appearance due to gliosis. Apart from these well-recognised changes there is usually increased visibility of the underlying choroidal vessels and there may be a diffuse pigment stippling of the fundus background. Many patients show a reduced visual acuity at an early stage and this may be associated with degenerative changes at the macula or with a curious reflex in the macula area.

A variety of fundus changes have been described in carriers of retinitis pigmentosa from scattered white spots to irregular pigmentation and the so-called tapetal reflex (Krill, 1967).

Other changes in the eye. Patients with retinitis pigmentosa quite commonly show posterior cortical lens opacities as the disease progresses and both glaucoma, myopia and macular degeneration have a significant genetic association. Along with myopia, vitreous detachment has also been shown to be relatively common, but there are several other intra-ocular changes described where the relationship with retinitis pigmentosa is less clear cut.

Dark adaptation and fields. An important early sign is the raising of the dark-adapted threshold to light. This can often be demonstrated simply by darkening the room and then assessing the patient's ability to find his way about after waiting ten minutes. For most clinical purposes the Goldman–Weekers dark adaptometer is one of the most useful ways of measuring these changes. The scotopic component of the dark-adaptation curve eventually disappears in more advanced cases so that the notch in the curve which is normally present disappears and the curve represents the adaptation to light of the cones only (Figure 8.1). Testing the visual field reveals a ring scotoma which often starts in the inferior temporal quadrant and spreads around the equatorial region.

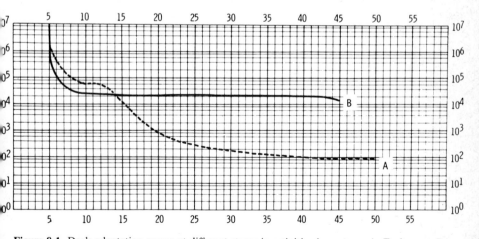

Figure 8.1. Dark-adaptation curves at different stages in retinitis pigmentosa. A. Early case. B. Advanced case. Adapted from Franceschetti, Francois & Babel (1963) *Les Heredo-dégénérescences Choriorétiniennes,* **1,** 226, Paris: Masson et Cie, with permission.

The field defect may then advance so that only a small central island of vision remains. In the dominant form of the disease the field defect more commonly begins in the far periphery so that a generalised constriction of the vision may be present from the start. On the other hand the ring scotoma is said to be more common in recessive cases (Krill, 1972). In sectorial retinitis pigmentosa, an atypical form where a sector of the retina only is involved the field defect is limited to that sector and may be bitemporal or hemianopic. The value of the electroretinogram in elucidating these unusual field defects will be discussed later.

Electrodiagnostic investigations in retinitis pigmentosa

When Karpe published his important paper on clinical electroretinography in 1945 he included five cases of retinitis pigmentosa in his section on 'electroretinography under pathological conditions'. All of these cases had an extinguished electroretinogram. He used an 8V lamp as stimulus with a shutter which gave flashes lasting 1/25 sec. The intensity of the continuous light could be adjusted to give between 1·25 and 80 lux at the eye. Since then, by using a stronger stimulus light and more sophisticated recording equipment, it has been shown that a selective impairment of the response may occur in the early stages and the amount of impairment depends to some extent on the genetic type of retinitis pigmentosa. The place of electro-oculography has also been explored and gross abnormalities occur at an early stage.

The electroretinogram in retinitis pigmentosa

At this point it may be helpful to remember that the electroretinogram and the electro-oculogram are two techniques designed to measure the changes of the resting or corneoretinal potential in response to light. The electroretinogram gives a measure of the brief changes which ensue after a single flash of light and the electro-oculogram measures the slow changes which occur when the eye is exposed to prolonged periods of light or darkness. The period of measurement for the electroretinogram is in the region of 400 msec and for the electro-oculogram it is half an hour. The electroretinogram is the most important of these tests at present for investigating retinitis pigmentosa, since it has been used much more extensively in the past. As a general rule the electroretinogram is affected at an early stage in the disease at a point when the fundus changes are minimal or absent (Figure 8.2). It is affected more severely in recessive cases where the prognosis is worse, whereas, relatively well-preserved responses may be found in dominant cases.

The relationship of the electroretinogram to the severity of the disease

In practice, most of the patients that one examines who show the typical fundus changes have an extinguished electroretinogram and it has been suggested that the response may be extinguished from birth (Franceschetti, Francois and Babel, 1963). However, using a technique which employed selective amplification, Henkes and co-workers showed that a photopic response could be recorded in four out of twelve typical cases when the electroretinogram as normally measured was unrecordable (Henkes, Van der Tweel and Van der Gon, 1956). It has also been shown that there is a close relationship between the electroretinogram sensitivity and the functioning area of the retina

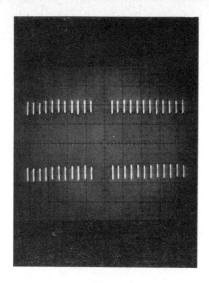

RETINITIS PIGMENTOSA

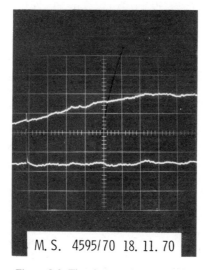

Calibration

400 μV

10 m. sec.

M. S.   4595/70   18. 11. 70

Figure 8.2. The electroretinogram and electro-oculogram in retinitis pigmentosa.

(Armington et al, 1961). It seems that when the electroretinogram is relatively well preserved the patients often give a history of a late onset and a mild form of the disease (Ruedemann and Noell, 1961). Table 8.1 shows a randomly selected series of 13 typical cases from the files of the Nottingham Electro-diagnostic Clinic. Five gave a dominant family history and eight were recessive. The electroretinogram was extinguished in all but two, one aged 64, the other 46.

Table 8.1. A series of unrelated patients showing the typical features of retinitis pigmentosa

Inheritance	Electroretinogram	Age	Severity
Dominant	Extinguished	15	Moderate
Dominant	Subnormal	46	Moderate
Dominant	Extinguished	23	Moderate
Dominant	Extinguished	64	Mild
Recessive	Subnormal	64	Severe
Recessive	Extinguished	50	Severe
Recessive	Extinguished	9	Severe
Recessive	Extinguished	22	Severe
Recessive	Extinguished	23	Severe
Recessive	Extinguished	27	Severe
Dominant	Extinguished	48	Moderate
Recessive	Extinguished	55	Severe
Recessive	Extinguished	40	Moderate

In some series where very early cases have been examined the electroretinogram has been almost normal and a very early change is usually seen in the scotopic electroretinogram, particularly if this is stimulated with a red light (Gouras and Carr, 1964). This type of abnormality has also been described in congenital stationary night blindness, but a distinction can be made between this relatively innocent condition and retinitis pigmentosa if one makes a careful measurement of the latencies of the components of the rod electroretinogram. Berson and co-workers have measured the latency and amplitude of the rod components of the electroretinogram using a blue stimulus in the dark-adapted state. They show a considerable delay in the responses of patients with dominant retinitis pigmentosa (Berson, Gouras and Gunkel, 1968). Therefore, either a red or a blue stimulus has proved useful in detecting early changes in the waveform of the response and in both instances the defect is seen in the rod response under dark-adapted conditions (see Chapter 7).

Rubino and Ponte published a collection of 30 cases of retinitis pigmentosa with a preserved electroretinogram in 1962. They divided these cases into two types: (1) those where the onset is late, the ophthalmoscopic and functional findings are mild and where the evolution is relatively slow; and (2) those which show an early onset in infancy or adolescence but have atypical fundus features and slow evolution. In some of these patients the fundus was normal and in almost all the persistence of the peripheral field with only a moderate ring scotoma was observed (Rubino and Ponte, 1962).

The relationship of the electroretinogram to the inheritance pattern

Electroretinography has served to confirm the value of a genetic classification of retinitis pigmentosa. In the recessive type the 'b' wave is practically always abolished whereas in the dominant type it may be present to some degree (Franceschetti, Francois and Babel, 1963). Krill mentions a type of recessive retinitis pigmentosa where the disease is mild and of late onset and in this rare type electroretinogram is relatively well preserved (Krill, 1972). Some recent studies in different families including a careful examination of very early cases have produced some interesting data. Berson and Kanters have shown a reduction in amplitude and an increase in latency of both rod and

cone responses of the electroretinogram in a family showing autosomal recessive inheritance (Berson and Kanters, 1970). On the other hand similar investigations in a family with dominantly inherited retinitis pigmentosa show loss
of rod function, but not of cone function in the early stages (Berson, Gouras
and Gunkel, 1968). The pattern of electroretinogram responses in patients
with sex-linked inheritance resembled that seen in the autosomal recessive
type. These electrodiagnostic studies of rod and cone function in early cases
entailed the use of scotopically balanced stimulus lights. The balance was
achieved by matching a short wavelength and a long wavelength light to produce equal subjective thresholds for normal dark-adapted subjects. Full-field
stimulation was used (Figure 8.3).

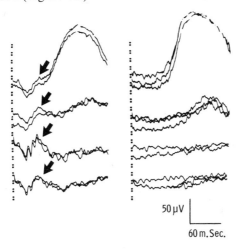

50 µV

60 m.Sec.

Figure 8.3. Shows suprathreshold responses to scotopically balanced red light (left-hand side),
and blue light (right-hand side) stimuli. Four different cases of increasing severity are represented
successively from top to bottom. All suffered from dominant retinitis pigmentosa and the early
cone component can be seen (arrowed) in the red light response in all cases, even though the rod
response is abolished in the lower two cases. Reproduced from Berson, E. L., Gouras, P. &
Gunkel, R. D. (1968) Rod responses in retinitis pigmentosa dominantly inherited. *Archives of
Ophthalmology*, **80**, 59–67. Copyright 1968 American Medical Association, with permission.

Detection of carriers. The electroretinogram can be used to detect early cases
of retinitis pigmentosa and considerable interest has also been focussed on the
possibility of detecting carriers in the sex-linked type. Krill examined four
carriers from three families and all showed some degree of fundus abnormality. Some showed scattered pigmentation and others showed a speckled golden
opacity in the macula area, the so-called tapetal reflex. Two of these carriers
are reported as having subnormal electroretinograms (Krill, 1967). There are
also other reports of abnormal electroretinograms in carriers of retinitis pigmentosa, but the observed changes are usually slight (Schappert-Kimmijser,
1963; Franceschetti, Francois and Babel, 1963; Kurstjens, 1965). A recent
study involved the examination of 91 members in five generations; five female
carriers were examined and all showed fundus abnormalities. In general the
carriers showed mild changes in visual function, including the electrical
responses, despite marked changes in the fundi (Imaizuni et al, 1972).

Other components of the electroretinogram

The early receptor potential might be expected to show interesting changes in retinitis pigmentosa because it is thought to be related to the bleaching of visual pigments in the outer segments of the rods and cones. Rather surprisingly, if one examines the human early receptor potential in retinitis pigmentosa, one finds that although it is reduced in amplitude it may be still present at a late stage in the disease (Table 8.2). The table shows that the early receptor potential was reduced below the normal mean amplitude of 220 μV in all cases except one, but sometimes the response may be abolished even though good central vision is preserved. There are various possible explanations for these discrepancies. One could assume that the preservation of the early receptor potential compared with the 'a' and 'b' waves at a late stage in the disease may be explained by a large cone component, these receptors being well preserved in some cases. It is also possible that the recording conditions in retinitis pigmentosa are markedly altered by the pathological changes themselves. Thus an electrical response may be present but not conducted to the recording equipment due to these physical alterations in the retina (see also Tamai, 1974).

Table 8.2. The early receptor potential in patients with retinitis pigmentosa

Age	Visual acuity	Early receptor potential (μV)	'a' and 'b' waves
20	6/18	80	Absent
21	6/12	0	Absent
25	6/18	0	Absent
28	Rt 6/9	360	Normal
	Lt 6/9	200	Reduced 'a' Absent 'b'
36	–	0	Absent
54	–	120	Reduced 'a' Absent 'b'
57	6/9	180	Reduced 'a' & 'b'
57	6/9	0	Absent
76	6/12	220	Reduced 'a' Absent 'b'

The early potential is usually reduced in value in patients with retinitis pigmentosa and it may be abolished when the visual acuity is still good.

Recovery of the early receptor potential. If one repeats the stimulus flash immediately after recording the early receptor potential, no response is obtained and it is necessary to wait for some seconds before it begins to reappear. In fact it does not reach its normal size again for several minutes. The rate of early receptor potential recovery has been correlated with the regeneration of visual pigments (Cone, 1964). It has been shown that in dominantly inherited retinitis pigmentosa the recovery rate is faster than normal (Berson and Goldstein, 1970a) (Figure 8.4). This abnormally rapid recovery rate may be partly due to the disappearance of the more slowly recovering rod response but may also be due to a more generalised abnormality of receptor function (Berson and Goldstein, 1972). Similar changes have been found in patients with sex-linked retinitis pigmentosa and in the female carriers a

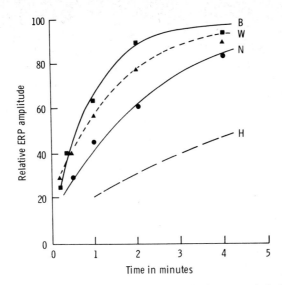

Figure 8.4. Average early receptor potential recovery rates for four normals (solid circles). Curves B and W represent recovery times in patients with dominant retinitis pigmentosa. Curve H is the recovery curve from a subject with hereditary rod monochromatism. Reproduced from Berson, E. L. & Goldstein, E. B. (1970) Average early receptor recovery rates. *Archives of Ophthalmology*, **83**, 418. Copyright 1970 American Medical Association, with permission.

reduction in amplitude of the early receptor potential was noted when the rod and cone electroretinogram was normal (Berson and Goldstein, 1970b; Berson, 1977).

The oscillatory wavelets. The literature concerning the fate of this component in retinitis pigmentosa is rather sparse, but examination of our own cases indicates that the size of the wavelets declines with the rest of the response. A small series of wavelets may sometimes be seen when the electroretinogram is still just detectable. Since there is evidence to suggest that this component is largely a photopic response (Jacobson, Hirose and Popkin, 1968), it is perhaps not surprising that it is not impaired at an early stage in retinitis pigmentosa.

The electro-oculogram in retinitis pigmentosa

The electro-oculogram, as assessed by the method of Arden and Kelsey (see Chapter 7), is very susceptible in primary pigmentary degeneration and this slow response to light may disappear completely at an early stage. Disputes have arisen as to whether the electroretinogram or the electro-oculogram is affected first; this would appear to depend on the accuracy of measurement in each case. When the photopic and scotopic components are examined carefully there is no doubt that very early electroretinographic changes can be detected (Gouras and Carr, 1964). However, in other series a marked reduction in the electro-oculogram is seen before the electroretinogram is seriously affected (Arden and Fojas, 1962). These authors have shown that the electro-oculogram light rise may be reduced when the dark-adaptation curve was near normal. In most cases the standing potential remains at a very steady level reminiscent of that seen in atrophic eyes. It is concluded that 'the finding of a flat electro-oculogram with the preservation of sufficient visual function to enable the patient to lead a normal life is pathognomonic of primary pigmentary retinal degeneration'. The electro-oculogram is therefore a useful test to perform on suspected cases of retinitis pigmentosa, especially as it is simpler to do than the electroretinogram. A contact lens is not required and the test can now be done by an unskilled assistant. However, we must bear in mind the fact that it is less easy to do accurate electro-oculography on a blind patient without fixation. The electroretinogram on the other hand does not require the patient to fixate accurately. In blind patients with retinitis pigmentosa one usually finds that not only is the light rise of the electro-oculogram absent, but the resting potential may be reduced; this is often immediately evident on examining the trace since the excursions are abnormally small.

Level of dark trough of electro-oculogram. As the disease advances the dark trough rises as the level of the light rise falls, but a resting potential is still evident in cases where the light rise and electroretinogram are absent. This has been termed the 'light-insensitive component' of the electro-oculogram. An ingenious method for assessing the light-insensitive component has been suggested. This depends on the presumed contribution of the corneal potential to the standing potential. In line with the theory that the corneal potential is abolished by the application of tetracaine drops to the cornea, it can be shown that an apparent sharp rise in the resting potential occurs after instilling these drops. This is because the corneal potential normally acts against the standing potential produced by the retina. Tetracaine drops were instilled into seven normal eyes and seven eyes with retinitis pigmentosa while the eye movement potential was being measured under constant illumination. The actual increase in potential caused by tetracaine treatment is almost the same in both instances since there is no corneal abnormality in retinitis pigmentosa; however the percentage increase in the potential is much greater in the latter than in the normals.

Although there are numerous studies of the electrical responses of female carriers in sex-linked retinitis pigmentosa, the unaffected heterozygous members of families with autosomal inheritance have had less attention. De Haas et al investigated three families with Usher's syndrome. Nine heterozygotes had abnormal electro-oculograms and two others showed doubtfully normal responses. They conclude that electro-oculography offers a diagnostic means for detecting the carrier state in relatives of an affected individual. However, normal values do not exclude the possibility of a patient being heterozygous. All these cases had normal electroretinograms (De Haas et al, 1970).

The relationship of the electrical response to the histological changes in retinitis pigmentosa

The histological changes in retinitis pigmentosa are characterised by progressive degeneration of the retinal receptors and subsequent general atrophy of the whole retina affecting first the outer and then the inner layers. In most of the cases where histological changes have been reported the condition has been at an advanced stage, but even in advanced cases it is possible to trace the course of the pathological process by referring to different parts of the retina. The changes may be summarised as follows:

1. A progressive atrophy of the sensory elements of the retina starting in external layers.
2. Alterations in the retinal and choroidal vasculature.
3. An active proliferation of the pigment epithelium.

In addition a thickening of the internal limiting membrane and a proliferation of the retinal glial tissue has been described (Franceschetti, Francois and Babel, 1963). Degenerated receptors may be more or less replaced by neuroglia. The ganglion cells and the nerve fibre layer remain unaffected until a late stage. The optic nerve may be completely atrophic or at other times relatively normal. In places there are gaps in the external limiting membrane and in these areas can be seen migration of pigment from the pigment epithelium into the sensory retina. Usually large clumps of pigment are visible, particularly around the veins.

Recent evidence suggests that the disease begins in the pigment epithelium. Even in early cases a widespread abnormality of the pigment epithelium can be demonstrated by fluorescein angiography (Krill, Archer and Newell, 1970). Early involvement of the electro-oculogram suggests early damage to the pigment epithelium and it has been shown in rats with retinitis pigmentosa that the pigment epithelium fails to perform its normal function. Normally the rods undergo a process whereby a portion of the structure is renewed and the old segment is taken up and phagocytosed by the pigment epithelium. In the diseased rats there is accumulation of these dead-rod outer segments and a breakdown of rod metabolism. This is an interesting observation but one must be very careful about drawing conclusions from analogous diseases in animals (Herron et al, 1969).

There are two ways of explaining the changes in the electroretinogram and the electro-oculogram.

1. The mode of production of the response may be altered. Because small electroretinograms may be recorded in patients whose dark adaptation is minimally affected and because correlations between field loss and electro-retinogram amplitude do not always hold in the early stage of the disease, one is bound to doubt that the electroretinogram is extinguished solely because the retinal sensitivity is depressed and a large area of the retina is non-functional. It seems likely that the functioning retina is itself producing an abnormal response and this is borne out by the changes seen in the early receptor potential.

2. Another way of explaining the changes would be to postulate that the disease process shunts out the electroretinogram current so that it cannot be picked up by the corneal electrode. This idea was suggested by Riggs in 1954, and Arden has further suggested that changes in Brindley's 'R' membrane may be responsible for this shunt (Arden and Fojas, 1962). The 'R' membrane is the resistive backing to the retina which was originally discovered by microelectrode techniques and the current flowing across this membrane causes the drop in voltage which is recognised as the electroretinogram in intraretinal recordings. The main part of the 'R' membrane is the inner bounding membrane of the pigment epithelium.

For more detailed reviews of retinitis pigmentosa the reader is referred to Landers et al (1977), Merin and Auerbach (1976) and Jay (1978).

The visually evoked response in retinitis pigmentosa

There is good evidence to show that the visually evoked reponse is largely a macular response. The cortical representation of the macular area is large compared with the representation of the peripheral fundus and good fixation of the stimulus light is necessary to obtain a maximal response. One might therefore expect little change in the visually evoked response in retinitis pigmentosa since macular function seems to be preserved to a late stage in the disease. In practice this appears to be the case. The visually evoked response is well preserved especially when a red-light stimulus is used and the response remains fairly good until a late stage (Nagaya and Hirata, 1967).

The Electroretinogram in Atypical Forms of Retinitis Pigmentosa

Sectorial retinitis pigmentosa

This condition was first described by Bietti in 1937 in a 25-year-old woman with symmetrical pigmentary changes in the inferior nasal quadrant of each eye. Numerous reports have been made since then and the distribution in the inferior nasal quadrant is the commonest form. In most cases the inheritance is autosomal dominant but it has been described as sex-linked recessive as well as autosomal recessive. In some families the other affected members have suffered from typical diffuse retinitis pigmentosa. A careful evaluation of three patients in 1970 (Krill, Archer and Newell, 1970) showed that all had a family history of retinitis pigmentosa, two with dominant inheritance and one recessive. Fluorescein angiography revealed changes corresponding with the involved sectors, but perimetric dark adaptation revealed more extensive involvement in some patients. Evidence of more widespread disease was confirmed in these cases by more severe electroretinogram changes. The electroretinogram is always subnormal in these patients but only very rarely has it been reported as extinguished (Figure 8.5).

Pasco reviews 24 case reports between 1937 and 1967 and concludes that this is a well-defined entity where the electroretinogram is always present but reduced. Most cases are mild and do not seem to progress, but some symmetrical cases appear to represent a form of classical retinitis pigmentosa evolving in the normal way (Pasco, 1970; Bisantis, 1971).

In another report of seven similar cases of sectorial pigmentary retinopathy, the authors consider that the disease is probably a very slowly progressive form of the more diffuse disease. In all these cases there was evidence of more widespread retinal involvement, and it is suggested that the apparently healthy retinal quadrants were probably potentially dystrophic. On the other hand the prognosis in these cases is comparatively good (Francois, De Rouck and Golan 1977).

SECTOR RETINITIS PIGMENTOSA

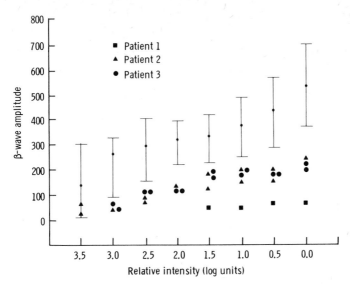

Figure 8.5. 'b' wave amplitudes in microvolts from three patients with sector retinitis pigmentosa and a normal control group. Reproduced from Krill, Archer & Martin (1970) Sector retinitis pigmentosa. *American Journal of Ophthalmology*, **69**, 983, with permission of authors and editor.

Unilateral retinitis pigmentosa

This condition has excited considerable interest in recent years and it is probably more common than the number of reported cases would indicate. Franceschetti, Francois and Babel laid down the following requirements for diagnosis:

1. Exclusion of inflammatory origin, in particular syphilis and viral infections.
2. Presence in the affected eye of symptoms typical for primary pigmentary degeneration.
3. Absence in the fellow eye of symptoms of tapeto-retinal dystrophy with the presence of a normal electroretinogram.

Many of the reported cases have certain features in common. They have no family history of relevant eye disease, and in some instances there are barely detectable changes in the fellow eye. For example the electro-oculogram may be at the lower limit of normal and there may be minimal pigment disturbance (Kolb and Galloway, 1964; Henkes, 1966) (Figure 8.6). There are two reasons why the diagnosis may be uncertain in all these cases; firstly it may be that the condition is bilateral but only one eye has so far been affected and the minimal changes sometimes noted in the fellow eye would support this, although the age of the patient often makes it unlikely. Secondly, the changes could all be post-inflammatory in spite of the diagnostic criteria laid down by Franceschetti et al. As an example we have seen two cases with a proven history of choroiditis and who apart from the history could not have been distinguished from the cases previously described by us in 1964.

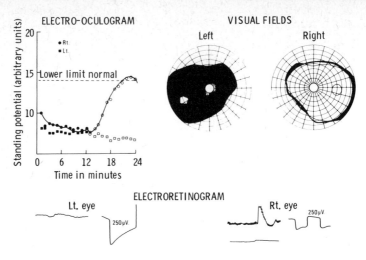

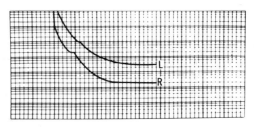

DARK ADAPTATION THRESHOLD

Figure 8.6. Electroretinogram, electro-oculogram, fields and dark adaptation in a case of unilateral retinitis pigmentosa. Reproduced from Kolb & Galloway (1964), *British Journal of Ophthalmology*, **48**, 473, with permission of authors and editor.

CASE 1. This patient was a male aged 60 years who presented with retinitis pigmentosa in his left eye only. This eye was aphakic and the lens had been removed following a perforating injury in his teens. The sight of his left eye had been poor since the injury and particularly in dim light. The left fundus, electrodiagnostic results and fields were all typical.

CASE 2. This patient, a middle-aged female, presented with severe unilateral choroiditis, the fundus being obscured by vitreous haze. All the routine investigations failed to reveal any systemic cause for this. The condition gradually cleared on local and systemic steroids and after some months a pigmented fundus could be seen with 'bone spicule' pigment and background changes resembling retinitis pigmentosa. Visual fields, dark adaptation and electrodiagnostic tests all mimicked unilateral retinitis pigmentosa.

The theoretical importance of this type of case is obvious. It seems that very occasionally inflammatory changes in the choroid can mimic retinitis pigmentosa very closely to the extent that they cannot be distinguished by electrodiagnostic or other clinical tests.

The Electroretinogram in Retinis Punctata Albescens

Retinitis punctata albescens is one of the progressive peripheral retina degenerations and it must be distinguished from a condition with similar features but which does not progress. This latter condition has been called the non-progressive form of retinitis punctata albescens or alternatively fundus albipunctatus. In practice there would appear to be some overlap between these two forms.

Examination of the fundus reveals diffusely scattered white dot-like lesions situated deep to the retinal vessels and associated with some impairment of night vision. It is usually congenital or begins at an early age and the high incidence of consanguinity indicates a recessive pattern of inheritance. Apart from the white dots in the fundus, the retinal vessels may be narrowed and there may also be scattered areas of pigmentation. In some patients the visual acuity is impaired and there may be construction of the visual fields. Abnormalities of colour vision have also been described.

Little is known about the nature of these white dots; they are more numerous at the posterior pole of the fundus and are thought to lie in the outer layers of the retina or the pigment epithelium. However, they have been described in the inner layers of the retina and even covering the retinal vessels (Bietti, 1942). Similar white dots are sometimes seen in otherwise typical cases of retinitis pigmentosa showing the close relationship between the two conditions.

The electroretinogram is usually completely abolished in these patients (Franceschetti, Francois and Babel, 1963), whereas it is preserved in the stationary form. An electrodiagnostic investigation is therefore of some value in these cases since it may indicate the prognosis. Problems arise, however, with intermediate forms which may show features of both the progressive and stationary types. Although there are many reports of an extinguished electroretinogram in retinitis punctata albescens, the point in the progress of the disease at which this occurs has not been clearly demonstrated. However, the close relationship of this condition with retinitis pigmentosa suggests that the electroretinogram may be affected at a very early stage, probably in infancy or even from birth (Jacobson, 1961; Marmor, 1977).

The Electroretinogram in Leber's Amaurosis

Leber's amaurosis was first described by Leber in 1869. He classed the condition with pigmentary degenerations of the retina even though the pigmentation was minimal or appeared at a late stage (Leber, 1869). The condition is usually congenital, the affected child being blind from birth; some cases become blind during the first year of life. The fundi may appear normal but a variety of minor changes have been described from fine pigment stippling to choroidal sclerosis (Franceschetti, Francois and Babel, 1963). On occasions the classical appearance of retinitis pigmentosa may be observed.

The advent of electroretinography has made it possible to distinguish these children from those with optic atrophy and Tay-Sachs disease. Since it is usually necessary to examine the fundi under a general anaesthetic it is important to take the opportunity to perform electroretinography at the same time. If a general anaesthetic is contra-indicated it is often surprisingly easy to insert a contact lens without an anaesthetic in a child up to three or four months old.

The absence of the electroretinogram in these cases was first stressed by Franceschetti and Dieterle (1954), and further interest was evoked when Schappert-Kimmijser and co-workers examined 113 eyes in a series of blind children. They found an absent response in 68 cases, using Karpe's technique, and these authors conclude that Leber's amaurosis affects 18 per cent of blind children (Schappert-Kimmijser, Henkes and Van der Bosch, 1959). It seems likely that the condition is much more common than has been supposed in the past and this may be because many cases pass out of the hands of the ophthalmologist once they have been labelled as blind. Thus clinical supervision may be lost before the diagnosis has been confirmed. Henkes has developed a technique for investigating the electro-oculogram under general anaesthesia and this has been applied to suspected cases of Leber's amaurosis. By assuming a pigment epithelium origin of the electro-oculogram he divides his cases into two groups:

1. Those with an absent electroretinogram but a normal or only slightly reduced electro-oculogram.
2. Those with an absent electroretinogram and an absent or grossly impaired electro-oculogram.

The patients in group 1 tended to show minimal fundus changes whereas those in group 2 showed more marked features of a tapeto-retinal degeneration. He concludes that Leber's amaurosis may include some cases with retinal dysgenesis which do not progress and others where there is a superimposed abiotrophy which show progressive changes, more marked fundus changes and gross electro-oculogram changes (Henkes and Verduin, 1963).

Leber's amaurosis is thought to have autosomal recessive inheritance and it may be associated with a variety of other conditions. Those within the eye include keratoconus, degeneration of the macula, cataract and chorio-retinal atrophy, but the patients are also often mentally defective and show congenital abnormalities elsewhere.

One would hope that in future years the combined use of the electroretinogram, the electro-oculogram and the visually evoked response will enable clinicians to distinguish with some confidence between those children where blindness is entirely due to retinal disease and those with occipital lobe damage.

Central Progressive Degenerations

Central Retinitis Pigmentosa

This condition has not been well defined in the past, but it is generally referred to as a variant of retinitis pigmentosa where the spider-like clumps of pigment are distributed around the macular area (Duke-Elder, 1967; Deutman, 1971). The term 'inverse retinitis pigmentosa' has been used, indicating the initial central field defect which tends to spread peripherally as opposed to the initial peripheral defect which spreads centrally in classical retinitis pigmentosa. Central retinitis pigmentosa must be distinguished from Stargardt's disease, vitelliform dystrophy and other conditions associated with pigmentation at the posterior pole.

The relatively few reports in the literature indicate the rarity of the condition but electroretinogram studies show a reduction of the photopic components at an early stage. Hommer showed these changes in a family, some members of which had central retinitis pigmentosa and some of whom showed the peripheral type (Hommer, 1969). The electro-oculogram has been described as initially normal but subnormal after some time (Deutman, 1971).

Progressive Cone Degeneration

In 1956 two articles appeared in the literature describing patients who experienced a progressive deterioration of visual acuity and yet in the initial stages the fundi appeared normal. It has of course been well recognised for many years that the ophthalmoscopic changes in the early stages of some types of macular degeneration may be very subtle. This is especially the case in children where the subjective assessment of the vision may be questioned. The important feature of these cases was the apparent selective damage to the cones, the rods being spared. Francois et al described a patient whose vision seemed worse in daylight; there were minimal fundus changes but evidence of extensive cone damage when the colour fields were plotted (Francois, Verriest and De Rouck, 1956). Steinmetz, Ogle and Rucker (1956) reported an autosomal dominant pedigree in which individuals showed an impairment of visual acuity, photophobia and defective colour discrimination years before macula degeneration became visible with the ophthalmoscope. Sloan and Brown described five patients with similar signs and symptoms. Three of these patients gave a family history of macula disease and four had photophobia. Examination of the visual fields showed a widespread involvement of the cones and the dark-adaptation curve was biphasic with a high cone threshold. These authors attempted electrodiagnostic investigations but concluded that 'currently used procedures for measuring the photopic electroretinogram may not be sensitive enough to detect the initial stages' (Sloan and Brown, 1962).

Since these earlier reports a considerable interest has been shown in the possibility of a pure cone disease and in theory at least the electroretinogram should be helpful in making the diagnosis. In fact it has now been shown that the flicker electroretinogram is particularly sensitive for this purpose (Goodman, Ripps and Siegal, 1964) (Figure 8.7).

Progressive cone dystrophy is now often considered as one entity in the wider group of 'cone dysfunction syndromes'. This group includes the congenital defects of colour vision and has been well defined by Goodman, Ripps and Siegal (1963). It is not easy to distinguish between stationary congenital achromatopsia and progressive cone degeneration without careful follow up. Both conditions may present with defective colour vision, subnormal vision and an absent electroretinographic response to a flickering stimulus. Nystagmus, photophobia and macular changes may also be present in both conditions. The history of progressive or stationary disease may be the only distinguishing feature. The electro-oculogram has been reported as normal in progressive cone degeneration (Goodman, Ripps and Siegal, 1964).

From these preliminary studies it seems clear that the electroretinogram has a useful place in elucidating macular degeneration, particularly in children

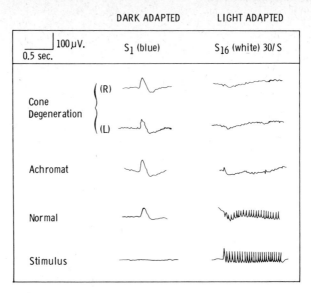

Figure 8.7. Electroretinogram recorded from the right and left eyes of a patient with progressive cone degeneration, a congenital achromat, and a normal subject. Note absence of flicker responses in all but normal. Reproduced from Goodman, Ripps & Siegel (1964) Progressive cone degeneration. *IIIrd ISCERG Symposium*, 365. Pergamon Press, with permission of authors and editor.

and in future the electroretinogram may be supplemented by the visually evoked response and the foveal electroretinogram. (Pearlman et al, 1974; Oguchi and van Lith, 1974).

Heredomacular Dystrophies

This includes a group of diseases characterised by bilateral macular degeneration, a hereditary tendency and the absence of associated disease in the central nervous system. These diseases have been classified and named eponymously according to the age of onset, but it has been suggested that they are all one and the same condition (Duke-Elder, 1967). They may be listed as follows:

Infantile heredomacular dystrophy—Best's disease or vitelline dystrophy.

Juvenile heredomacular dystrophy—Stargardt's disease.

Adult heredomacular dystrophy—Behr's disease.

Presenile and senile heredomacular dystrophies.

As a general rule these patients present with a gradual deterioration of their central vision. In children there may be difficulty in reading or seeing the blackboard at school, which is not corrected by wearing glasses. The fundus appearance varies considerably from case to case; in Best's disease a round or oval lesion is seen at the macula which has a yellowish colour and has been likened to the yolk of an egg—hence the term 'vitelline dystrophy'. The vitelline lesion evolves into a pigmented scar. Rather surprisingly the vision of these patients may remain normal in spite of the fundus appearances. In Stargardt's disease, which usually appears between the ages of eight years and eleven years, the vision may be impaired when the fundus is still normal. The earliest change is disappearance of the normal foveal reflex and grey, yellow or brown spots may appear at the macula. Eventually an oval circle of pigment stippling is seen and occasionally this may spread to involve the entire posterior pole in rare cases. Senile macular degeneration is associated with degenerative changes in the underlying choroid and Bruch's membrane, and although it may bear some resemblance to the types which occur at an earlier age, it may be complicated by the presence of haemorrhages and subretinal exudates. Sometimes senile macular degenerations are divided into dry and wet types, or the degeneration of Haab, and disciform degeneration respectively (Gregor, Bird and Chisholm, 1977).

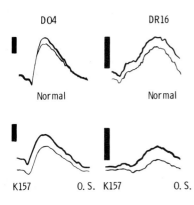

Figure 8.8. The electroretinogram in heredomacular degeneration. Normal response above, responses to red light on right. Note: (a) change in shape of 'a' wave; (b) loss of 'a' wave and 'x' wave in lower red response. Reproduced from Ruedemann, A. D. (1969) Electroretinogram in heredomacular degeneration. *International Ophthalmology Clinics*, **9**, 1020. Boston: Little, Brown, with permission of author and editor.

Electrodiagnostic investigations

It has been shown that if the macular area in the monkey is photocoagulated then the electroretinogram obtained from this damaged eye is quite normal (Jacobson, Najac and Stephens, 1960). Furthermore, a normal electroretinogram has been described in cases of solar retinopathy (Ponte, 1961). It is not surprising therefore that early reports reveal normal electrical responses in these cases (Karpe, 1945; Dollfus, Krauthamer and Chalvaignac, 1951). However when examination is carried out using a red light stimulus a high percentage of cases show a reduced amplitude of the 'b' wave (Jacobson, Basar and Kornzweig, 1956; Jayle, Boyer and Camo, 1959). The photopic electroretinogram has also been shown to be normal but Jaegar, Lux and Grutzner (1961) showed that the spectral sensitivity curve of the photopic electroretinogram may be displaced towards the shorter wavelengths. Ruedemann and Noell examined five cases of macular degeneration using their own strict protocol. This entailed varying the stimulus intensity of a Grass stroboscope, using red and blue filters, investigating the response to flicker and recording the results on Polaroid film from the face of an oscilloscope. In all these cases the electroretinogram showed an overall reduction in amplitude, a reduction and blunting of the flicker response, a reduced 'x' wave in response to red light and poorly developed 'humps' on the 'b' wave (Figure 8.8). They claim that

changes can be seen on the electroretinogram if the degenerate area is larger
than one disc diameter (Ruedemann and Noell, 1961). Niemayer has also
shown a significant reduction in the 'b' wave amplitude in 22 eyes with juvenile
macular degeneration and 45 eyes with senile macular degeneration. He found
that the photobic 'b' wave in red light was specifically reduced in juvenile
cases and that the electrical changes were not proportional to the visual loss
or the ophthalmoscopic findings (Niemayer, 1969). The apparent discrepancies
in the various reports on macular degeneration would seem to be largely due
to differences in technique. It seems likely that as more sophisticated methods
are used, more and more abnormalities will be found. Recently Stangos et al
measured the averaged photopic electroretinogram in macular degeneration:
80 per cent of 239 eyes gave an abnormal response. They showed that using a
weak red stimulus, 66 per cent of the 'dry' type and nearly all the cases of
disciform degeneration were abnormal (Stangos, Spiritus and Korol, 1972).

The foveal electroretinogram has also been shown to be subnormal in all
cases including those in which the visual acuity was still fairly good (Figure
8.9). The visually evoked response has also been shown to be abnormal
(Bankes, 1967; Deutman, 1971).

Some slightly unexpected changes have been described in the electro-oculogram in cases of macular degeneration. Several different sources report that
the electro-oculogram may be markedly impaired as the sole sign of disturbed
retinal function in patients with vitelline dystrophy. The electroretinogram in
these cases is usually normal (Krill et al, 1966; Francois, De Rouck and
Fernandez-Sasso, 1966). In Stargardt's disease the electro-oculogram is
usually normal unless there is involvement of the retinal periphery (Neetens
et al, 1977).

It is therefore no longer true to say that the electroretinogram and the
electro-oculogram are normal in patients with macular degeneration, but the
difficulty still remains that a physically minute lesion can cause a serious
disturbance of vision where macular disease is concerned. Thus one would
expect to find relatively minor changes in the electrical responses even with
quite severe impairment of visual acuity. The foveal electroretinogram is a
very promising technique but its value is limited when opacities in the media
scatter the stimulus light and the use of averaging techniques and a weak red
stimulus may be more helpful in these cases.

Progressive Degeneration Associated with Choroidal Degeneration

Choroideremia

Choroideremia is a rare congenital condition of some theoretical importance
from the genetic point of view. The inheritance pattern is intermediate sex
linked so that only males are affected and all the daughters of affected males
are heterozygous carriers. The female carriers transmit the disease to 50 per
cent of their sons and show characteristic non-progressive fundus changes.

The main symptoms in the affected males are night blindness and progressive contraction of the visual fields. Although the condition is usually congenital, contraction of the visual fields may not appear until the teens, and
blindness does not occur until the age of 35 or 40. In childhood the fundus
may show peripheral degeneration of the pigment epithelium and areas where

LEFT DISCIFORM MACULAR DEGENERATION

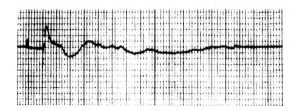

Left Eye V. A. 6/60

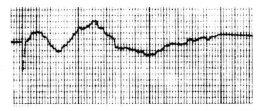

Right Eye V. A. 6/9 Normal

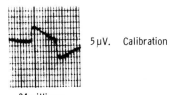

5 μV.   Calibration

34 millisecs.

Figure 8.9. Foveal electroretinogram shows reduction in peak to trough amplitude. Foveal electroretinogram of the right eye is normal and shown for comparison. Reproduced from Bankes, J. L. (1967) *The Foveal Electroretinogram. Transactions of the Ophthalmic Society of the United Kingdom*, **87**, 255, with permission of the Council.

the choroidal vessels are exposed. Gradually the retina and choroid become extensively atrophic so that by the age of 50 the whole sclera may be exposed, leaving a small island of relatively normal fundus in the central area.

In the female carriers the fundus shows peripheral pigment stippling resembling the appearance seen in affected males in early childhood. However, in the carriers the condition does not progress.

Electrodiagnostic investigations

Although the response of the electroretinogram is severely impaired, the photopic components are better preserved than in cases of retinitis pigmentosa. Pameyer and co-workers have observed a rudimentary response in a 58-year-old patient. Franceschetti, Francois and Babel also report a 'b' wave of 40 μV in a 40-year-old patient. In some early cases an 'a' wave alone has been recorded (Pameyer, Waardenburg and Henkes, 1960; Franceschetti, Francois and Babel, 1963).

In most cases the electroretinogram is normal in female carriers but minor abnormalities have been recorded. Pameyer described a diminished scotopic response and subnormal electroretinograms have been recorded in elderly patients. Jacobson and Stephens found that the 'b' wave did not increase in amplitude during dark adaptation in one case (Francois and De Rouck, 1958; Jacobson and Stephens, 1962). McCulloch notes that five female carriers out of the large family that he examined all had normal electroretinograms (McCulloch, 1969).

Gyrate Atrophy

This term refers to a striking change which may be seen in the peripheral fundus in early life. There are irregular white areas where the retina and choroid appear to have been punched out. In some areas the larger choroidal vessels may be preserved and there is a variable amount of pigment dispersion. Autosomal inheritance as a recessive trait is the rule and this distinguishes these cases from patients with choroideremia.

The areas of chorio-retinal atrophy extend and coalesce so that eventually the whole fundus may be involved. The fundus picture may therefore closely resemble that of choroideremia. However, unlike choroideremia most cases of gyrate atrophy are high myopes and in addition there is a high incidence of cataracts.

The progress of the disease is usually extremely slow and this is reflected in the electrical responses. Initially the patients become night blind and then a ring scotoma develops. Sometimes other members of the same family may be affected not by gyrate atrophy but by typical retinitis pigmentosa, thus demonstrating the relationship between the two conditions.

An interesting development in our knowledge of this condition has recently occurred. The majority of patients show a markedly increased plasma level of the amino acid ornithine. This may be increased to as much as ten times the normal level and although plasma levels in unaffected relatives are normal, the heterozygotes may be detected by means of a loading test (Takki and Simell, 1974).

Although there are only a limited number of reports on the results of electrodiagnostic tests, it would appear that the electroretinogram is relatively well preserved in the early stages and this is our own experience in the case of a female aged 18 years in whom the changes were limited to the peripheral fundus. Bourquin and Bourquin (1949) described a very early case with minimal fundus involvement and a normal electroretinogram. The response diminishes as the condition advances so that absent electroretinograms have been reported in some cases (Franceschetti and Dieterle, 1957).

Choroidal Sclerosis

The words 'choroidal sclerosis' refer to a fundus appearance in which there is baring of the choroid and prominence of the choroidal vessels. These vessels appear sclerosed but it is possible that true sclerosis is not present and the appearance is only due to the absence of the pigment epithelium.

Choroidal sclerosis may be seen in the fundi of patients with retinitis pigmentosa and there is undoubtedly some overlap between these conditions. It is usual to divide choroidal sclerosis into two types, a peripheral type and a central type.

Peripheral choroidal sclerosis

A generalised atrophy of the choroid begins to become apparent during the third or fourth decade. This gradually progresses so that the end result resembles that seen in choroideremia. Both dominant and recessive inheritance have been described and the field defect and abnormalities of dark adaptation may resemble retinitis pigmentosa. In the few cases described the electroretinogram has been markedly affected, being either subnormal or extinguished (McKay and Spivey, 1962; Franceschetti, Francois and Babel, 1963).

Central choroidal sclerosis

In this type the onset is at a similar age. The degenerate area at the posterior pole gradually takes on a pathognomonic appearance when a sharply defined circular or oval area of areolar atrophy develops in which the pigment epithelium and choriocapillaris have disappeared. Subjective symptoms may be delayed but eventually a central scotoma appears. The electroretinogram is usually normal but a 'b' wave of only 20 μV has been reported in one instance (Francois, Verriest and De Rouck, 1956, quoted in Franceschetti, Francois and Babel, 1963).

Sorsby's Pseudo-inflammatory Dystrophy

Sorsby described this heredo-degenerative dystrophy in 1949. The main features are the appearance of oedema, haemorrhages and exudates in the macular area of both eyes. This leads to a more generalised choroidal atrophy and the prognosis for vision is usually poor. Most cases show an autosomal dominant inheritance pattern. In the cases examined the electroretinogram has been well preserved and so it would appear that so far electrodiagnostic tests do now show any prognostic value in this condition. It is not usually possible to make a diagnosis of Sorsby's pseudo-inflammatory dystrophy by examining the fundus alone. The important diagnostic features are: (1) the bilateral symmetry of the lesions; (2) the absence of optic atrophy or alterations of the retinal vessels and the presence of a normal dark-adaptation curve and a normal electroretinogram; and finally (3) dominant inheritance.

Myopic Chorio-retinal Degeneration

Degenerative myopia is generally regarded as a separate entity from simple myopia. Whereas simple myopia is thought to be a normal variant in the biological series which includes emmetropia and hypermetropia, degenerative myopia is thought to be a pathological condition of unknown cause which may be related to the general group of inherited retinal degenerations.

Degenerative myopia generally shows a dominant pattern of inheritance but some cases appears to be related to prematurity or may follow toxaemia of pregnancy (Gardiner and James, 1960). The main clinical features are a combination of a highly myopic refraction, chorio-retinal degeneration and atrophy, thinning of the posterior sclera and an increased axial length of the eye. Although rare cases are congenital, it usually takes many years to develop and early cases cannot be distinguished from simple myopia.

Electrodiagnostic investigations

Karpe (1945) was the first to show that the electroretinogram may be subnormal in high myopes; three out of the four cases that he examined were subnormal and the remaining case was probably subnormal. Since then there have been numerous reports, most of which indicate a decline in amplitude of both photopic and scotopic components with progress of the myopia. Some authors have suggested that the electroretinogram changes may precede the ophthalmoscopic changes (Francois and De Rouck, 1955). Jayle and co-workers found an initial impairment of the photopic response but photopic and scotopic components were affected when the vision became impaired (Jayle, Boyer and Camo, 1959). In an investigation of 92 myopes, Dhanda has shown that the size of the 'b' wave is inversely proportional to the extent of degenerative changes and he suggests that an abnormally low potential may indicate an impending retinal detachment (Dhanda, 1966). In another more recent paper, a depression of the electroretinogram in myopic eyes with normal fundi seemed to indicate a trend towards pathological myopia (Malik et al, 1969). Ponte found that in simple myopia the mean amplitude of the 'b' wave was slightly reduced while in severe myopia the electroretinogram was markedly affected, the most common finding being a negative type of electroretinogram. The presence of a negative type of electroretinogram with a large 'a' wave in these patients has also been shown by Blach et al. They have investigated 35 patients with degenerative myopia and Figure 8.10 shows the types of waveform that they recorded. The electroretinogram amplitudes for 'a' and 'b' waves is also shown (Blach, Jay and Kolb, 1966). They also performed electro-oculograms on these patients: the mean electro-oculogram ratio was 176 per cent compared with a normal mean of 238 per cent. It is of interest that they found no correlation between the size of the light rise of the electro-oculogram and the degree of refractive error. This could simply reflect the rather wide range of values that are obtained in this type of investigation but may be due to the fact that all but four of their cases had more than eight dioptres of myopia. Those patients with abnormal dark adaptation and those with more severe degenerate changes tended to have lower light rises. Franceschetti reported little change in the electro-oculo-gram, but it is important to realise that he was using a completely different technique. This involves measuring the dark trough and not the light rise and so markedly different results might be expected (Franceschetti, Francois and Babel, 1963). In a carefully documented series of 16 patients of a family suffering from nyctalopia with myopia, Völker-Diben et al found that the EOG was almost normal in all cases. In general the electrodiagnostic findings indicated that the receptor system was functioning normally. The wavelets tended to be absent in these cases and they concluded that most of the pathological disturbance in the retina must occur central to the receptors (Völker-Diben, et al, 1974).

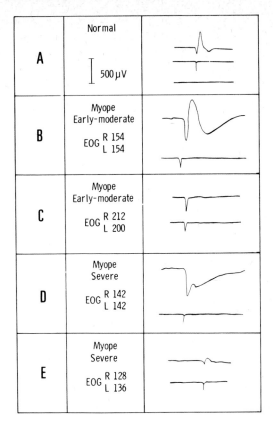

A	Normal $\mathbf{I}$ 500 µV	
B	Myope Early-moderate EOG R 154 L 154	
C	Myope Early-moderate EOG R 212 L 200	
D	Myope Severe EOG R 142 L 142	
E	Myope Severe EOG R 128 L 136	

Figure 8.10. The electroretinogram waveform in the early to moderate myope can vary from supernormal (B) to negative (C). In the severe myope the waveform can be negative with an enlarged 'a' wave (D) to minute (E). Reproduced from Blach, R. K., Jay, B. & Kolb, H. (1966) *British Journal of Ophthalmology*, **50**, 635, with permission of authors and editor.

Relationship between clinical appearance and pathological findings

Table 8.3 shows a summary of these relationships. It is certainly striking that the electro-oculogram changes parallel those seen in the pigment epithelium, but it is not quite so easy to explain the enlarged 'a' wave on existing theory and animal work. If we assume that the 'a' wave has increased because of a reduction in the size of the PII component of Granit (1933), then we must search for an early pathological change at the site of this component. This component is thought to arise from the region of the bipolar cells and yet changes in the inner retina occur late in myopia. This discrepancy will have to be explained by future work.

Table 8.3. Relationship between clinical appearance, pathological findings, and results of electrical tests in degenerative myopia

Clinical appearance	Changes in pigment epithelium	Changes in rods and cones	Changes in inner retina	EOG	ERG	Dark adaptation
Normal	n	n	n	n	n	n
Early	*	n	n	*	n	n
Early/Moderate	*	n	n	*	a+	n
Moderate	**	*	n	**	a+ b−	n
Moderate/Severe	***	*	n	***	a** b−	*
Severe	***	***	*	***	a * b−	**

*Slight abnormality   **Definite abnormality   ***Gross abnormality

Reproduced from Blach, R. K., Jay, B. and Kolb, H. (1966) Electrical activity of the eye in high myopia. *British Journal of Ophthalmology*, **50**, 640, with permission of authors and editor.

Angioid Streaks of the Retina

This interesting condition was originally described by Doyne in 1889, and ophthalmologists for many years thought that the remarkable appearance was due to haemorrhages or vascular abnormalities. It was not until 1929 that Groenblad and Strandberg related the fundus appearance to the skin condition known as pseudoxanthoma elasticum, and later it was also found in certain cases of Paget's disease and in sickle-cell disease (Groenblad, 1929). In 1935 Böck demonstrated histologically that the fundus appearance was due to ruptures in Bruch's membrane. Other changes in Bruch's membrane were also described and the whole picture is thought to be due to a more generalised defect of elastic tissue (Böck, 1935).

The fundus appearance is most commonly seen in association with pseudoxanthoma elasticum as the Groenblad–Strandberg syndrome. Brownish sinuous lines are seen which can be mistaken for abnormally large but rather indistinct blood vessels. Sometimes they are quite faint and difficult to see. There is a tendency for macular haemorrhages to occur and these may be preceded or followed by macular degeneration.

Electrodiagnostic investigations

A condition which involves selective damage to any layer of the retina is of particular interest to the electrodiagnostician. In this case the defect is in a layer which has been shown to have special importance in animal work. Microelectrode work suggests that Bruch's membrane, or the tissue immediately adjacent to it, has a high electrical impedance across which the electroretinogram is measured. Gaps in this membrane might therefore be expected to produce abnormalities of the response which were disproportionate to the amount of functional defect. However, according to most reports the electroretinogram is normal in the early stages and only becomes abnormal if the disease extends to the macular area (Francois and Verriest, 1954). Mazza and Molinari (1967) confirm that the standard response of the electroretinogram is normal, but they find an alteration in the response to red stimuli and a reduction in the threshold of the critical fusion frequency. (These findings are

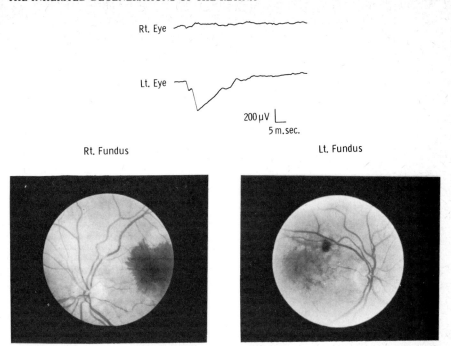

Figure 8.11. The electroretinogram and angioid striae. Note the grossly impaired response in the right eye. Although a disproportionate reduction of the electroretinogram might be expected in this condition, it is unusual.

merely indicative of the associated degeneration of the macula.) Figure 8.11 illustrates the case of a 40-year-old female with angioid streaks and pseudo-xanthoma elasticum. The striking feature is the grossly impaired response in the right eye compared with the left. The visual acuity was 6/9 in each eye, but she had suffered a large haemorrhage at the posterior pole of the right eye. Ophthalmoscopically the angioid streaks appeared equally extensive in the two eyes. The electro-oculogram showed a reduced light rise in both eyes. The right eye shows the type of response that one might see in retinitis pigmentosa (and it would be interesting to know if the response recovers in these patients when the haemorrhages have absorbed).

Progressive Degenerations of the Retina Associated with Vitreous Degeneration

These conditions may be divided into three main types, each of which shows a different mode of inheritance:

1. Juvenile sex-linked retinoschisis.
2. Autosomal recessive vitreo-retinal dystrophy (Goldmann–Favre disease).
3. Dominant vitreo-retinal dystrophy (Wagner's disease).

The first-mentioned is relatively common and the remaining two are rare. All types show degenerative changes in the retina and vitreous in young people, the main feature being a splitting of the inner layers of the retina to form what at first sight may be a localised retinal detachment. Sometimes the affected part of the retina has a cystic appearance but in other cases the retinoschisis may be more diffuse. At the posterior edge of the area of schisis or along its upper margin may be seen a line of pigment sometimes known as the 'high water mark', and oval openings, sometimes of considerable size, may be seen in the outer undetached layer of the retina.

Although there is similarity between all three conditions, the recessive and dominant types tend to show more degenerative changes in the vitreous with peripheral condensations and the formation of white strands in relation to the area of schisis. In these two conditions also there is more frequently associated night blindness and changes in the choroid and retina suggesting the hereditary pigmentary degenerations. The ultimate prognosis is poor and eventually a retinal detachment may develop, but the progress of the disease may be very slow.

Electrodiagnostic investigations

According to Franceschetti et al who quote Ricci (1961), the electroretinogram is subnormal in juvenile sex-linked retinoschisis but not to the extent that would be seen in a retinal detachment of the same extent. The electroretinogram is also subnormal in the dominant form. On the other hand, in the recessive type the electroretinogram tends to be abolished. However, this evidence appears to be based on the results from only a small number of cases (Franceschetti, Francois and Babel, 1963). A subnormal electroretinogram has been recorded on many occasions in juvenile sex-linked retinoschisis and Deutman confirms this in 26 cases. The electro-oculogram results published by the same author are interesting in that 15 out of 21 cases had a normal light rise, although they shows a subnormal electroretinogram. This indicates that the outer layers of the retina remain intact at least in the first instance. The situation is the reverse of that found in vitelline dystrophy where a grossly disturbed electro-oculogram is accompanied by a normal electroretinogram.

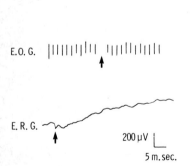

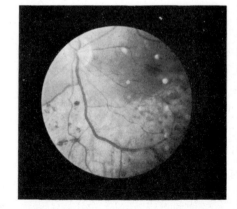

Figure 8.12. Favre's disease in a young girl showing marked reduction of the electroretinogram and abolition of the electro-oculogram light rise, despite a normal visual acuity and involvement of about the lower quarter of the retina. The other eye showed minimal changes.

Figure 8.12 shows the results obtained from a patient who had noticed blurring of her vision for about two years and on examination was found to have an area of retinoschisis in the inferior 1/4 of the retina of the left eye and minimal but similar changes in the periphery of the right eye. The electrical responses from the right side were normal, but quite severe impairment of the response from the left eye can be observed. The flat electro-oculogram is in contrast to the findings of Deutman in juvenile sex-linked retinoschisis.

Progressive Degenerations of the Retina Associated with Systemic Disease

A wide variety of diseases has been associated with retinitis pigmentosa and some of the other progressive degenerations mentioned above. Although in their present state of development electrodiagnostic investigations cannot distinguish between classical retinitis pigmentosa and that associated with disorders in the rest of the body, they have a particular value when applied to the latter. Sometimes the fundus changes are minimal in these patients and they may be referred from the neurologist or the physician with the question 'Are eyes normal?'. The electroretinogram and electro-oculogram can provide an immediate answer. Apart from this the vision may be affected by other pathological processes. Figure 8.13 shows the result from a patient with ill-defined peripheral constriction of her visual fields and enlargement of the pituitary fossa. She also had polydactyly, having had the extra fingers removed in infancy. The fundi showed one or two irregular flecks of pigment in the periphery. The problem was to decide whether the field defect was due to chiasmal compression or to early retinitis pigmentosa in association with polydactyly, the Laurence-Moon-Biedl syndrome being suspected.

A list of the systemic disorders associated with progressive retinal degeneration includes the following conditions:

    1. Metabolic disorders:
        a. Lipid abnormalities:
            i. A-beta-lipoproteinaemia
            ii. Refsum's disease
            iii. Familial amaurotic idiocy

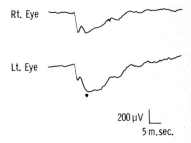

Figure 8.13. The electroretinogram in a patient with primary amenorrhoea, enlargement of the pituitary fossa, polydactyly, and 'non-specific' pigmentation of the fundus. There was also temporal constriction of the visual fields. The electroretinogram would suggest that her field defect was due to chiasmal compression rather than associated retinitis pigmentosa.

Rt. Eye

Lt. Eye

200 μV

5 m.sec.

2. Neurological disorders:
    a. Laurence-Moon-Biedl syndrome
    b. Hereditary ataxias
    c. Ocular myopathy
    d. Syndromes involving mental retardation

3. Occasional associations;
    a. Dermatological disorders
    b. Megacolon
    c. Marfan's syndrome
    d. Familial nephropathies

Most of the listed conditions are associated with retinitis pigmentosa, but familial amaurotic idiocy, although characterised by progressive degeneration of the retina, is probably a completely separate entity. The electroretinogram in the infantile form has been reported as normal from several sources and this in keeping with the pathological changes which at first are restricted to the ganglion cell layer and spare the outer parts of the retina whence the electroretinogram arises. In late infantile and juvenile amaurotic idiocy the electroretinogram may be reduced or absent, however (Copenhaver and Goodman, 1960). All the other conditions listed are associated with retinitis pigmentosa and the electroretinogram and the electro-oculogram are affected accordingly. The main interest of these other conditions is that several of them show specific biochemical abnormalities which seem to throw some light on the cause of the pigmentary degeneration. For example, the association of a-beta-lipoproteinaemia, retinitis pigmentosa, ataxia and acanthocytosis of the red cells (the Bassen–Kornzweig syndrome) also involves a lowering of the blood level of the fat-soluble vitamins including vitamin A. Recently it has been claimed that vitamin A supplements in sufficient dosage to raise the vitamin A level to normal will also lead to restoration to normal of the dark-adaptation curve and also the electroretinogram (Carr, 1970). In the muco-polysaccharidoses the vision may be impaired by infiltration of the cornea and the fundus may not be visible. Electrodiagnostic tests may thus be the only way of detecting associated retinitis pigmentosa.

Related Stationary Conditions

These may be classified into those conditions exhibiting night blindness and those where the dark adaptation is normal:

Non-Progressive Retinal Degenerations

1. Associated with night blindness
    a. Congenital night blindness with normal fundi
    b. Fundus albipunctatus
    c. Fundus flavimaculatus
    d. Oguchi's disease
    e. Congenital fleck retina

2. Without night blindness
    a. Congenital grouped pigmentation
    b. Sjögren's reticular dystrophy

Congenital night blindness with normal fundi may be inherited as dominant, sex-linked recessive, or autosomal recessive traits. Characteristic electroretinogram changes have been described in authentic cases. As one might expect, the scotopic element of the 'b' wave may be completely absent (Figure 8.14). In fact, the electroretinogram changes may closely resemble those seen in very early cases of retinitis pigmentosa. However, it has been shown recently that the latency is increased in retinitis pigmentosa, whereas it is normal in congenital stationary night blindness (Berson et al, 1969; Carr, 1969).

Fundus albipunctatus refers to a condition resembling retinitis punctata albescens and it is sometimes termed the stationary form of retinitis punctata albescens; it can be distinguished by the normal electroretinogram (Francois, Verriest and De Rouck, 1956), normal retinal vessels and visual acuity and a mild form of night blindness.

Fundus flavimaculatus is characterised by the appearance of white spots in the retina scattered around the posterior pole, but in this case the visual function including electroretinogram and dark adaptation is normal.

Oguchi's disease is a congenital functional defect of the rod system with recessive inheritance. Most of the known cases have been described from Japan. The rather remarkable feature of this condition is the fundus appearance which changes with dark adaptation. The light-adapted fundus has a grey/white colour and this gradually changes to a normal colour after dark adaptation. Dark adaptation is abnormally slow and may take as long as three hours. The visual acuity and fields are normal. The changes in the electroretinogram have been described as follows:

After five minutes dark adaptation a negative response is obtained with a white flash stimulus of 80 lux. Flicker fusion occurs at 20/sec instead of at 30–35/sec at this level of dark adaptation. After dark adaptation the response remains unchanged for at least half an hour. The scotopic 'b' wave is usually absent and the 'a' and 'x' waves are well developed. The tendency towards a negative response can help to distinguish this type of electroretinogram from that sometimes seen in fundus albipunctatus (Francois, Verriest and De Rouck, 1956).

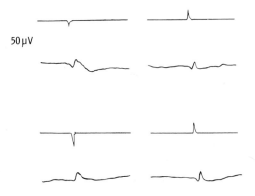

50 µV

Figure 8.14. On the left: normal electroretinogram showing photopic and scotopic 'b' wave. On the right: the rod component is absent in a patient with congenital night blindness. Reproduced from Franceschetti, Francois & Babel (1963) *Les Heredo-dégénérescences Choriorétiniennes*, **II**, 1214, Paris: Masson et Cie, with permission.

Congential grouped pigmentation and Sjögren's reticular dystrophy both show normal electrical responses and neither condition is associated with any functional defect of vision.

SUMMARY

The recording and interpretation of the electroretinogram has advanced considerably since the publication of Karpe's now classical paper in 1945. It is still recognised that as a general rule the electrical response is severely impaired in all the true hereditary retinal degenerations, with the exception of Tay-Sachs disease and those conditions in which the disease process is strictly limited to the macula area. However, since the earliest cases were reported in the 1940s it has been possible to examine patients at a much earlier stage in the disease process and to show that the rod components in the electroretinogram are first affected. The electro-oculogram is also affected at a very early stage. It is possible that careful studies of alterations in the latency of the response will also help us to reach a firm diagnosis in some cases; further diagnostic evidence may be provided by measuring the recovery time of the early receptor potential. It is becoming evident therefore that not only changes in amplitude, but also changes in the pattern of the waveform, can provide the clinician with information on patients with inherited degenerations of the retina.

REFERENCES

Arden, G. B. & Fojas, M. R. (1962) Electrophysiological abnormalities in pigmentary degenerations of the retina. *Archives of Ophthalmology*, **68**, 369–389.
Armington, J. C., Gouras, P., Tepas, D. & Gunkel, R. (1961) Detection of the electroretinogram in retinitis pigmentosa. *Experimental Eye Research*, **1**, 74–80.
Bankes, J. L. K. (1967) The foveal electroretinogram. *Transactions of the Ophthalmological Society of the United Kingdom*, **67**, 249–262.
Berson, E. L. (1977) Hereditary retinal diseases: classification with the full-field electroretinogram. *Documenta Ophthalmologica* (Proceedings Series) **13**, 149.
Berson, E. L. & Goldstein, E. B. (1970a) Average early receptor recovery rates. *Archives of Ophthalmology*, **83**, 418.
Berson, E. L. & Goldstein, E. B. (1970b) The early receptor potential in sex linked retinitis pigmentosa. *Investigative Ophthalmology*, **9**, 58–63.
Berson, E. L. & Goldstein, E. B. (1972) Cone pigment degeneration, retinitis pigmentosa and light deprivation. *Vision Research*, **12**, 749–752.
Berson, E. L., Gouras, P. & Gunkel, R. D. (1968) Rod responses in retinitis pigmentosa dominantly inherited. *Archives of Ophthalmology*, **80**, 58–67.
Berson, E. L., Gouras, P., Gunkel, R. D. & Myrianthopoulos, N. (1969) Rod and cone responses in sex linked retinitis pigmentosa. *Archives of Ophthalmology*, **81**, 215.
Berson, E. L. & Kanters, L. (1970) Cone and rod responses in a family with recessively inherited retinitis pigmentosa. *Archives of Ophthalmology*, **84**, 288–297.
Bietti, G. (1942) Fondo puntato albescente con emeralopia congenita e sindatillia familiare. (Contributo alla conoscenza delle forme atipiche di sindrome di Lawrence-Blodi e della morfologia delle chiazette del fondo oculare). *Bollettino d'Oculistica*, **21**, 636–650.
Bisantis, C. (1971) Sectorial pigmentary retinopathy of G. Bietti. *Annales d'Oculistique*, **204**, 907–954.
Blach, R. K., Jay, B. & Kolb, H. (1966) Electrical activity of the eye in high myopia. *British Journal of Ophthalmology*, **50**, 629–641.
Böck, J. (1935) Zwei Schwestern mit gefässähnlichen Netzhautstreifen und Pseudoxanthoma elasticum der Haut. *Klinische Monatsblätter für Augenheilkunde*, **44**, 691–692.

Bourquin, J. & Bourquin, J. B. (1949) À propos d'une atrophia gyrata choroideae et retinae de Fuch's apparaissant dans une famille de retinites pigmentaires. *Ophthalmologica*, **118**, 848–857.

Carr, R. E. (1969) The night blinding disorders. *International Ophthalmology Clinics*, **9** (4), 971–1003.

Carr, R. E. (1970) Vitamin A therapy may reverse degenerative retinal syndrome. *Clinical Trends in Ophthalmology, Otorhinolaryngology and Allergy*, **8**, 8.

Cone, R. A. (1964) Early receptor potential of the vertebrate retina. *Nature*, **204**, 736–739.

Copenhaver, R. M. & Goodman, G. (1960) The electroretinogram in infantile, late infantile and juvenile amaurotic idiocy. *Archives of Ophthalmology*, **63**, 559–566.

De Haas, E. B. H., Van Lith, G. H. J., Rijnders, J., Rumke, A. M. L. & Völmer, C. (1970) Usher's Syndrome: With special reference to heterozygous manifestations. *Documenta Ophthalmologica*, **28**, 166–190.

Deutman, A. F. (1971) *The Hereditary Dystrophies of the Posterior Pole*, **6**, 189–197. Assen: Royal Van Gorcum.

Dhanda, R. P. (1966) Electroretinogram and dark adaptation study in myopic retinal degeneration. *Proceedings of the All-India Ophthalmic Society*, **23**, 77–82. (Published 1968).

Dollfus, M. A., Krauthamer, S. & Chalvaignac, A. (1951) Sur un nouvel appareil d'électrorétinographie et premiers résultats cliniques. *Bulletin des Sociétés d'Ophthalmologie de France*, **51**, 627–635.

Donders, F. C. (1855) Torpeur de la rétine congénitale héréditaire. *Annales d'Oculistique*, **34**, 270–273.

Duke-Elder, Sir Stewart (1967) *A System of Ophthalmology*, **10**, 574. London: Henry Kimpton.

Falls, H. F. & Cotterman, C. W. (1948) Choroidoretinal degeneration: A sex-linked form in which heterozygous women exhibit a tapetal-like retinal reflex. *Archives of Ophthalmology*, **40**, 685.

Franceschetti, A. & Dieterle, P. (1954) L'importance diagnostique et pronostique d'électrorétinogramme dans les dégénérescences tapéto-rétiniennes avec rétrissément du champ visual et hemeralopie. *Confinia Neurologica*, **14**, 184–186.

Franceschetti, A. & Dieterle, P. (1957) Die differential diagnostische Bedentung des ERG bei tapetoretinalen degenerationen. *Bibliotheca Ophthalmologica*, **48**, 161–181.

Franceshcetti, A., Francois, J. & Babel, J. (1963) *Les Héredo-dégénérescences Chriorétiniennes*, **1**, 226–306. Paris: Masson.

François, J. & De Rouck, A. (1955) L'électrorétinographie dans la myopie et les décollements myopigenes de la retine. *Acta Ophthalmalmologica*, **33**, 131–155.

François, J. & De Rouck, A. (1958) L'intérêt de l'électrorétino-encéphalographie dans le diagnostique differential dégénérescences tapéto-rétiniennes. *Bulletin de la Société Belge d'Ophthalmologie*, **117**, 511–538.

François, J., De Rouck, A. & Fernandez-Sasso, D. (1966) L'électro-oculographie dans les kystes vitelliformes de la macula. *Bulletin de la Société Belge d'Ophthalmologie*, **143**, 547–552.

François, J., De Rouck, A. & Golan, A. (1977) ERG in sectorial pigmentary retinopathy. *Documenta Ophthalmologica* (Proceedings Series), **13**. 239.

François, J. & Verriest, G. (1954) Les fonctions visuelles dans le lastose rétinienne. *Annales d'Oculistique*, **197**, 113–144.

François, J., Verriest, G. & De Rouck, A. (1956) Les fonctions visuelles dan les dégénérescences tapéto-rétiniennes. *Bibliotheca Ophthalmologica*, **43**, 22–26.

Gardiner, P. A. & James, G. (1960) Association between maternal disease during pregnancy and myopia in the child. *British Journal of Ophthalmology*, **44**, 172–178.

Goodman, G., Ripps, H. & Siegel, I. M. (1963) Cone dysfunction syndromes. *Archives of Ophthalmology*, **70**, 214–231.

Goodman, G., Ripps, H. & Siegel, I. M. (1964) Progressive cone degeneration. *Proceedings of the 3rd Symposium of ISCERG*, pp. 363–372. (Ed.) Burian, H. & Jacobson, J. H. London: Pergamon.

Gouras, P. & Carr, R. E. (1964) Electrophysiological studies in early retinitis pigmentosa. *Archives of Ophthalmology*, **72**, 104–109.

Graefe, A. Von (1858) Exceptionelles Verhalten des Gesichtsfeldes bei Pigmententartung der Netzhart. *Graefes Archiv für Ophthalmologie*, **4** (II), 250–253.

Granit, R. (1933) The components of the retinal action potential in mammals and their relation to the discharge in the optic nerve. *Journal of Physiology*, **77**, 221.

Gregor, Z., Bird, A. C. & Chisholm, I. H. (1977) Senile disciform macular degeneration in the second eye. *British Journal of Ophthalmology*, **61**, 141–147.

Groenblad, E. (1929) Angioid streaks—Pseudoxanthoma elasticum: vorläufig Mitteilung. *Acta Ophthalmologica*, **7**, 329.

Henkes, H. E. (1966) Does unilateral retitinitis pigmentosa really exist. An electroretinogram and electro-oculogram study of the fellow eye. In *Clinical Electroretinography* (Ed.) Burian, H. M. & Jacobson, H. H. *Proceedings of 3rd Symposium of ISCERG. Visual Research Supplement*. London: Pergamon.

Henkes, H. E., Van der Tweel, L. H. & Denier Van der Gon, J. J. (1956) Selective amplification of the electroretinogram. *Ophthalmologica*, **132**, 140–150.

Henkes, H. E. & Verduin, P. C. (1963) Dysgenesis or abiotrophy? A differentiation with the help of the electroretinogram and the electro-oculogram in Leber's congenital amaurosis. *Ophthalmologica*, **145**, 144–160.

Herron, W. L., Riegel, B. W., Myers, O. E. & Rubin, M. L. (1969) Retinal dystrophy in the rat— a pigment epithelial disease. Investigative Ophthalmologica, **8**, 595–604.

Hommer, K. (1969) Das Elektroretinogramm bei der zentralen Retinitis pigmentosa. *Albrechte von Graefes Archiv für klinische und experimentelle Ophthalmologie*, **178**, 30–43.

Imaizumi, K., Takahashi, P., Tazawa, Y., Yamada, K. &. Mita, K. (1972) Clinical and electro-physiological observations on genetic carriers of retinitis pigmentosa in a family (pedigree Tt) showing sex-linked inheritance. *Advances in Experimental Medicine and Biology*, Vol. 24, London: Plenum.

Jacobson, H. J. (1961) Retinitis punctata albescens. In *Clinical Electroretinography*, pp. 108–113. Springfield, Illinois: Thomas.

Jacobson, J. H., Basar, D. & Kornzweig, A. L. (1956) Spectrod-differential electroretinography in macula disease. *American Journal of Ophthalmology*, **42**, (II), 199–205.

Jacobson, J. H., Hirose, T. & Popkin, A. B. (1968) Independence of the oscillatory potential, photopic and scotopic b-waves of the human electroretinogram. In *The Clinical Value of Electroretinography. ISCERG Symposium* (Ghent), pp. 8–20. Basel/New York: Karger.

Jacobson, J. H., Najac, H. T. & Stephens, G. (1960) The role of the macula in the electroretinogram of monkey and man. *American Journal of Ophthalmology*, **50**, 889–899.

Jacobson, J. H. & Stephens, G. (1962) Choroideretinal degeneration. Sex-linked inheritance. *Archives of Ophthalmology*, **67**, 321–335.

Jaeger, W., Lux, P. & Grutzner, P. (1961) Subjektiv und objectiv spektrale Helligkeitsverteilung bei angeboren und erworbenen Farbensinnstörungen. In *Neurophysiologie und Psycophysik des Visuellen Systems*. (Ed.) Jung, R. & Kornhuber, H. pp. 199–209. Berlin: Springer.

Jay, B. (1978) Prevention of blindness from retinitis pigmentosa. *Transactions of the Ophthalmological Society of the United Kingdom*, **98**, 309–311.

Jayle, G. E., Boyer, R. L. & Camo, R. L. (1959) *L'électro-retinographie Dynamique en Ophthalmologie*. Paris: Masson.

Karpe, G. (1945) The basis of clinical electroretinography. *Acta Ophthalmologica*. Supplement **24**.

Kolb, H. & Galloway, N. R. (1964) Three cases of unilateral retinitis pigmentosa. *British Journal of Ophthalmology*, **48**, 471–479.

Krill, A. E. (1967) Observations of carriers of X-chromosomal linked chorioretinal degeneration. *American Journal of Ophthalmology*, **64**, 1029–1040.

Krill, A. E. (1972) Retinitis pigmentosa: a review. *Sight Saving Review*, **42**, 21–28.

Krill, A. E., Archer, D. & Martin, D. (1970) Sector retinitis pigmentosa. *American Journal of Ophthalmology*, **69**, 977–987.

Krill, A. E., Archer, D. & Newell, F. W. (1970) Fluorescein angiography in retinitis pigmentosa. *American Journal of Ophthalmology*, **69**, 826–835.

Krill, A. E., Morse, P. A., Potts, A. M. & Blein, B. A. (1966) Hereditary vitelliruptive macular degeneration. *American Journal of Ophthalmology*, **61**, 1405–1415.

Kurstjens, J. H. (1965) Choroideremia in gyrate atrophy of the choroid and retina. *Documenta Ophthalmologica*, **19**, 1.

Landers, M. B., Wolbarsht, M. L., Dowling, J. E. & Laties, A. M. (1977) (Eds) Retinitis pigmentosa: clinical implications of current research. In *Advances in Experimental Medicine and Biology*. New York: Plenum Press.

Leber, Th. (1869) Ueber Retinitis pigmentosa und angeboren Amaurose. *Graefes Archiv für Ophthalmologie*, **15**, (III), 1–25.

Malik, S. R. K., Gupta, A. K., Gupta, P. C. & Singh, G. (1969) Electroretinogram in myopia. *All-India Ophthalmological Society*, **17**, 48–51.

Marmor, M. F. (1977) Defining fundus albipunctatus. *Documenta Ophthalmologica* (Proceedings Series), **13**, 227.

Mazza, C. & Molinari, I. (1967) Indagine elettroretinografica nell strie angiodi della retina. *Rivista Oto-Neuro-Oftalmologica*, **42**, 119–129.

McCulloch, C. (1969) Choroideremia: a clinical and pathological review. *Transactions of the American Ophthalmological Society*, **67**, 142–195.

McKay, R. H. & Spivey, B. E. (1962) Generalised choroidal angiosclerosis. *Archives of Ophthalmology*, **67**, 727–735.

Merin, S. & Auerbach, E. (1976) Retinitis Pigmentosa. *Survey of Ophthalmology*, **20**, 303–346.

Nagaya, T. & Hirata, A. (1967) Visual function test with electrophysiological methods. *Folia Ophthalmologica Japonica*, **18**, 126–131.

Neetens, A., Schneider, H., Van Elsen, E. & Janssens, M. (1977) Using electro-oculography and angiofluography for early diagnosis of the retino-choroidal diseases of the posterior pole. *Annales d'Oculistique* (Paris) **210**, 193–202.

Niemayer, G. (1969) Elektroretinographie bei Macula-degenerationen. *Albrecht von Graefes Archiv für klinische und experimentelle Ophthalmologie*, **177**, 39–51.

Oguchi, Y. & Van Lith, G. H. M. (1974) Contribution of the central and the peripheral part of the retina to the VECP under photopic conditions. *Documenta Ophthalmologica* (Proceedings Series), **4**, 261.

Pameyer, J. K., Waardenburg, P. J. & Henkes, H. E. (1960) Choroideremia. *British Journal of Ophthalmology*, **44**, 724–738.

Pasco, M. (1970) Sectorial symmetrical pigmentary degeneration of the retina. *Archives d'Ophthalmologie*, **30**, 481–486.

Pearlman, J., Owen, W. G., Brounley, D. W. & Sheppard, J. J. (1974) Cone dystrophy with dominant inheritance: post clinical case histories. *Documenta Ophthalmologica* (Proceedings Series), **4**, 123.

Ponte, F. (1961) Electroretinography in solar macular injury. *1st Symposium of ISCERG (Stockholm)*. *Acta Ophthalmologica*, **70**, 238–244. (Published 1962).

Ricci, A. (1961) Clinique et transmission héréditaire des dégénérescences vitreorétiniennes. *Bulletin des Sociétés d'Ophthalmologie de France*, **61**, 618–662.

Riggs, L. A. (1954) Electroretinography in cases of night blindness. *American Journal of Ophthalmology*, **38**, 70–78.

Rubino, A. & Ponte, F. (1962) The role of electroretinography in the diagnosis and prognosis of retinitis pigmentosa. *Acta Ophthalmologica*, **70**, 232–237.

Ruedemann, A. D. (1969) The electroretinogram in heredomacular degeneration. *International Ophthalmology Clinics*, **9**, 1020.

Ruedemann, A. D. & Noel, W. K. (1961) Electroretinogram in central retinal degeneration. *Transactions of the American Academy of Ophthalmology and Otolaryngology*, **65**, 576–594.

Schappert-Kimmijser, J. (1963) Les dégénérescences tapéto-rétiniennes du type X-chromosomal aux Pays-Bas. *Bulletin des Sociétés d'Ophthalmologie de France*, **76**, 122–129.

Schappert-Kimmijser, J., Henkes, H. E. & Van der Bosch, J. (1959) Amaurosis congenita (Leber). *Archives d'Ophthalmologie*, **61**, 211.

Sloan, L. & Brown, D. J. (1962) Cone dysfunction syndrome. *American Journal of Ophthalmology*, **54**, 629–641.

Stangos, N., Spiritus, M. & Korol, S. (1972) Electroretinogram and electro-oculogram in macula degeneration. *Archives d'Ophthalmologie*, **32**, 277–290.

Steinmetz, R. D., Ogle, K. N. & Rucker, C. W. (1956) Some physiologic considerations of hereditary macular degeneration. *American Journal of Ophthalmology*, **42**, 304–319.

Takki, K. & Simell, O. (1974) Genetic aspects in gyrate atrophy of the choroid and retina with hyperornithaemia. *British Journal of Ophthalmology*, **58**, 907–921.

Tamai, A. (1974) Studies on the early receptor potential in the human eye. III. ERP in primary retinitis pigmentosa. *Yonago acta medica*, **18**, 18–29.

Volker Dieben, H. J., Van Lith, G. H. M., Went, L. N. & De Vries De Mol, E. C. (1974) Electro-ophthalmology of a family with X chromosomal recessive nyctalopia and myopia. *Documenta Ophthalmologica* (Proceedings Series), **4**, 169.

CHAPTER NINE

The Value of Electrodiagnostic Investigations in Acquired Retinal Disease

In this chapter it is proposed to consider the electrical responses of the human eye in a variety of acquired diseases of the retina. Perhaps the greatest value of these tests is seen in conditions associated with opacities of the media, because in these cases the ophthalmoscope may not be of any help. A considerable amount of research is still being done on this subject, but at present it is clear that attempts at making specific diagnoses are often doomed to failure due to the diffuse nature of the response and our relative ignorance as to the significance of the different components that it displays. However, there is no doubt that in many instances additional information about the patient can be discovered. Sometimes this has prognostic value, sometimes diagnostic, but the electroretinographer's dream of fitting the electrodes, pressing the stimulus button, and reading off the diagnosis from an illuminated panel is far removed from reality with our present state of knowledge.

Much systematic work has been carried out on the subject of retinal detachment and more recently there has been an upsurge of interest in diabetic retinopathy. The changes seen in the various vascular retinopathies have also been explored and these, together with the inflammatory diseases, will also be considered. Finally, it is important to consider those conditions involving the optic nerve and ganglion cells which may cause serious disturbance of the retina. The visually evoked response is now proving useful in distinguishing these, and it should always be used to investigate patients in whom the vision is poor and the electroretinogram is normal.

ELECTRODIAGNOSIS AND RETINAL DETACHMENT

The term retinal detachment refers to a state of separation of the sensory retina from the pigment epithelium which is almost invariably irreversible in man, and results in degeneration of the sensory elements of the retina in the absence of surgical treatment. Effective surgical treatment became available in the 1920s when it was discovered that a cure could sometimes be effected by sealing the small holes in the retina which accompany retinal detachment. Since then several important advances have been made and modern methods can produce a good visual result in up to 80 per cent of cases. However, every surgeon still experiences tragic cases where blindness ensues after surgery has been repeated many times. It is in the early detection of these cases that the electroretinogram may play a part and in particular in assessing the future prospects of the fellow eye. When the presence of opacities in the media prevents an accurate assessment of the extent of the detachment, the electro-retinogram may also be of considerable value.

Preliminary studies of the electroretinogram in retinal detachment were made in 1948 (Karpe, 1948), and it soon became apparent that it is associated with a marked diminution in amplitude of the 'b' wave. The change in the electrical response probably occurs immediately, coinciding with the loss of visual function (Figure 9.1); the retina must therefore be against the pigment epithelium if it is to produce a normal response in the human. Several articles appeared in the 1950s dealing with limited numbers of cases, but a more thorough investigation was reported by Francois and De Rouck in 1955. They examined 26 cases but in only two of these could pre- and post-operative results be compared. In one of these surgery was successful in spite of an extinguished electroretinogram (Francois and De Rouck, 1955). Schmöger also reported cases where successful surgery was associated with an extinguished electroretinogram and did not feel that the electroretinogram could provide any help in the prognosis of retinal detachment (Schmöger, 1957). However, since then several authors have expressed a contrary view about this (Asayama et al, 1957; Jacobson et al, 1958). A detailed and extensive study of many aspects of this subject has been reported by Rendahl (1961). Most of this work has been done using methods similar to those described by Karpe and attention has been concentrated largely on the size of the 'b' wave.

Table 9.1. Relationship of size of 'b' wave to extent of detachment

Results	I n	b-pot. mean	mV s	II n	b-pot. mean	mV s	III n	b-pot. mean	mV s	IV n	b-pot. mean	mV s
Op. successful (group A)	16	0·22	0·08	47	0·15	0·07	11	0·07	0·05	1	0·00	—
Op. unsuccessful (group B)	44	0·15	—	18	0·09	0·06	13	0·03	0·04	2	0·00	—
No op. (group C)	11	0·09	—	14	0·12	0·08	3	0·03	—	24	0·01	0·02

See text for definition of groups. Reproduced from Rendahl (1961) *Acta Ophthalmologica*, **24**, 64, with permission.

A distinct relationship between the size of the 'b' wave and the extent of the detachment has been shown to exist in all the larger published series. Table 9.1 shows the results obtained by Rendahl. The extent of the detachment is indicated by dividing the cases into groups. Group I included patients

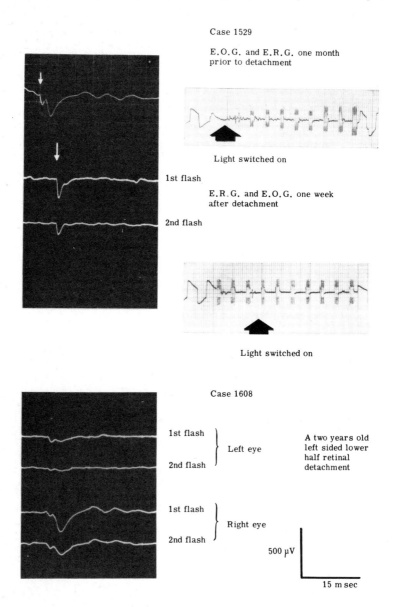

Figure 9.1. Electro-oculography before and after the occurrence of a detachment. The electro-oculogram was recorded fortuitously prior to the detachment because the other eye was being investigated.

with less than a quarter of the retina detached, Group II with between a quarter and a half of the retina detached, Group III with between one half and three quarters detached, and Group IV had subtotal detachments where more than three quarters of the retina was detached. It can be seen that the 'b' wave is gradually diminished with increasing extent of the detachment.

Relationship of the Size of the 'b' Wave to the Cause of the Detachment

There does not appear to be any significant difference in the reduction of the size of the 'b' wave when different aetiological groups are considered, although the response from the fellow eye tends to be normal in patients with idiopathic detachment. Myopic patients also tend to show a reduction in size of the 'b' wave in the absence of a retinal detachment and it is important to take this fact into account when considering the results. It has been claimed that retinal detachment due to the presence of a malignant tumour produces a disproportionate impairment of the response in some cases. This may be due to infiltration of the retina beyond the detached region (Sundmark, 1958).

The Effect of Pre-operative Bedrest on the Response

It is interesting that Rendahl examined the electroretinogram of several patients when they were being treated with pre-operative bedrest. Serial recordings from these patients showed an improvement of the response in a few cases as the retinal detachment decreased in extent. In most instances however the response did not seem to alter; the follow-up results on these patients suggest that a pre-operative improvement of the response may have a particularly favourable prognosis (Rendahl, 1961).

The Electroretinogram and the Prognosis in Retinal Detachment

At first sight it seems helpful to make a statistical analysis of the results of retinal detachment surgery and to compare these with the results of pre-operative electroretinograms and indeed, by these means, it has been shown that the size of the electroretinogram is related to the result of surgery. Parizot summarises this as follows:

1. If the 'b' wave is larger than 200 μV a surgical success is the rule with a good visual acuity.
2. If the size of the 'b' wave lies between 175 μV and 200 μV good results are still obtained in most cases.
3. If the 'b' wave is below 100 μV a functional result may be obtained in about 50 per cent of cases.
4. If the electroretinogram is extinguished then the best result that can be expected is a flat retina with poor central acuity (Parizot, 1967).

The problem is to decide whether this is achieving any more than an assessment of the prognosis in terms of the extent of the area of retina detached. There are already several well-recognised prognostic features such as the site and size of the retinal tears, and these include the extent of the detachment. We do not yet know for certain whether the electroretinogram shows anything more than simply the size of the detached area and if this is the case its value would be limited to patients with opaque media. When the media are clear the extent of the detachment can be conveniently measured by perimetry, although one must remember that electrodiagnostic tests have the great theoretical advantage of being completely objective. There is a little evidence to indicate that the electroretinogram also reflects predisposing degenerative features in the retina and several authors conclude that its prognostic value is not limited to an assessment of the area of the retina detached. This evidence is derived from investigations of the fellow 'healthy' eye.

The Electroretinogram in the 'Healthy' Eye

Rendahl has shown in a series of 102 cases that a lower mean value for the 'b' wave was present in the fellow eye of unsuccessfully treated patients compared with those who had had successful surgery. Myopic eyes were excluded from this series but similar findings were made in a group of myopic patients. About 20 per cent of cases of retinal detachment become bilateral, but we have yet to prove that a poor response in the fellow eye can indicate potential bilateral cases even though it may seem reasonable to suspect this. In fact some electrophysiological evidence now suggests that abnormalities may be found in the response from the good eye regardless of the fundus appearance (Tamai, 1977).

Other Components of the Response in Retinal Detachment

The light rise of the electro-oculogram is minimal or absent when more than 35 per cent of the retina is detached (Blach and Behrman, 1967; Lobes, 1978). The response is abolished as soon as the detachment occurs and may take up to a year to reach its former value after successful surgery. The size of the 'b' wave has also been noted to be small after successful surgery at least in the immediate post-operative period. It is interesting that the visual acuity may also recover very slowly; some of my own cases have shown an improvement of central vision during the course of the second post-operative year.

   Since the retinal as opposed to the choroidal circulation is preserved in retinal detachment, one might expect some selective loss of the components of the electroretinogram, those arising in the inner half of the retina being relatively well preserved. In fact a more generalised depression of retinal function seems to occur and in most cases the oscillatory potential is also impaired (Parizot, 1967).

   Yonemura et al studied the oscillatory potential in 19 cases of idiopathic detachment. They measured the sum of the amplitudes of the upward or positive deflections (ΣO) and compared this with the sum of the amplitudes of the negative or downward deflections (ΣN) and they concluded that: (1) ΣO was below the lower limit of the normal range in all 19 cases and ΣN was normal in two cases and subnormal in 17; (2) the peak latencies of the first positive and negative peaks were increased in about three quarters of the cases; (3) a reduction of the value of ΣO and ΣN was noted in about half of the fellow eyes. Some of the fellow eyes with abnormal oscillatory potentials showed peripheral chorio-retinal degeneration (Yonemura et al, 1972b).

   Although changes in the 'a' wave have not been extensively studied, it seems significant that Asayama found that whereas the 'b' wave remained impaired after successful detachment surgery, the 'a' wave showed good restitution to its presumed original value: Granit's PIII component appears to show an early recovery when the normal anatomy is restored.

The early receptor potential can still be seen when the retina is detached although its amplitude is reduced. It may persist when the other components of the electroretinogram have been completely abolished and it has been produced in longstanding detachments. However, it is rarely seen if the detachment has been present for some years (Figure 9.2). Since it is becoming recognised that some sight may be regained from treating longstanding cases by modern surgical techniques, the early receptor potential may be of some value in such patients (Galloway, 1970), as part of their pre-operative assessment. Table 9.2 shows some post-operative results as examples of the type of response that can be obtained using a bright stimulus flash. It can be seen that in one case the response did not recover in spite of successful replacement of the retina.

In a study of fellow eyes, it has been shown that 22 out of 41 eyes showed no appreciable retinal abnormalities, yet there was a significant decrease in the amplitude of the ERP. In the 19 fellow eyes that showed degenerative changes, including peripheral retinal breaks, the mean ERP amplitude showed a greater and highly significant decrease compared with a series of normal controls (Tamai, 1978).

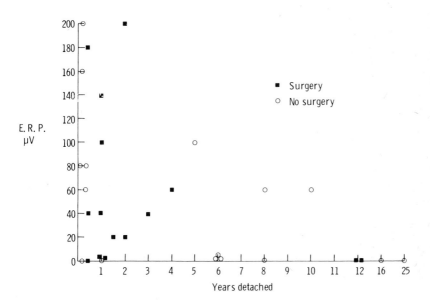

Figure 9.2. The ERP in total detachment.

Table 9.2. The response after successful surgery

Age	E.R.P. (μV)	a Wave (μV)	a-b Diff.* (μV)	Time Elapsed Since Surgery
50	100	80	100	*1 month*
50	180	140	200	*1 year*
37	0	0	0	*4 months*
38	R 60	180	240	*2 years*
	L 120	80	80	*1 year*

* a-b Diff. = difference in amplitude of a-b waves measured from peak to peak.

Retinal Detachment where the Fundus View is Obscured

Sometimes in elderly people it is difficult to assess the function of the retina behind a mature cataract and the presence of a retinal detachment can be excluded by electroretinography before considering surgery. Not uncommonly a retinal detachment may be associated with a vitreous haemorrhage. These patients are often treated with bed rest as a safety measure when the diagnosis is in doubt. Although an electroretinogram cannot with certainty exclude a flat retinal tear, it can confirm the presence of a detachment in these cases. In patients with a history of congenital cataract the fear of retinal detachment in middle life is always present and quite often it is difficult to examine the fundus when residual lens capsule occupies the pupil space. In such cases the electroretinogram may also provide helpful information for the surgeon.

Summary

The electroretinogram can undoubtedly provide useful information in patients with retinal detachment; it may give an objective assessment of the extent of the detachment and it may indicate the presence of degenerative changes in the other eye. The electroretinogram is of particular value in cases where there are opacities of the media and this applies especially to cases of vitreous haemorrhage where an associated retinal detachment is suspected. Middle-aged patients with congenital cataracts which were treated surgically in infancy also pose a diagnostic problem which can be solved by electroretinography. In these patients it is often very difficult to see the fundus through the small gap in the lens capsule and the risk of retinal detachment is high.

ELECTRODIAGNOSIS AND DIABETIC RETINOPATHY

It has been known for many years that the classical waves of the electroretinogram are not affected until a late stage in diabetic retinopathy and even then the reduction in amplitude does not show any features which might be specific for diabetes. However, a renewed interest in the subject was created by Yonemura, Aoki and Tsuzuki (1962) who described the selective disappearance of the oscillatory potential. Similar changes were also described in some other circulatory disturbances of the retina. Amongst other series published since then, Kurachi described an absent or diminished oscillatory potential in 24 out of 43 patients who had diabetes but no visible fundus changes (Kurachi et al, 1966). In 1966 Simonsen also described a diminution in the oscillatory potential in diabetics with normal fundi (Simonsen, 1966). A recent report involving a large series of eyes has shown beyond doubt that this component of the electroretinogram may be absent when a response recorded by the classical technique may be perfectly normal. Furthermore, there is no doubt that early changes are seen in diabetic retinopathy. The exact point in the development of the retinopathy at which the wavelets are affected differs markedly in different series but this is probably due to differences in stimulus parameters (Tassy, Jayle and Gastaut-Maysou, 1971). These authors examined 213 eyes in diabetic patients and compared the classical waveform with the oscillatory potential. The 'a' and 'b' waves did not show significant changes until stage III (Scott's classification—Scott, 1953). On the other hand a significant reduction of the oscillatory potential was seen in stage II and in some cases abnormalities were present before the development of the retinopathy. Changes in the wavelets were more evident in the dark-adapted state. In 1972 Yonemura calculated the sum of the amplitudes of the positive components of the wavelets (ΣO) in 172 diabetic eyes. He showed that the ΣO was significantly diminished in 31·5 per cent with stage O retinopathy, 62·5 per cent of eyes with stage I retinopathy, 60 per cent of eyes with stage II retinopathy, and 81·8 per cent with stage III retinopathy (Scott's classification). In the majority of cases the peak latency of the first wavelet was also increased and so this also appears to be a sensitive change (Yonemura et al, 1972a).

Individual Fundus Features and the Oscillatory Potential

In a recent study, a series of 30 patients (60 eyes) was examined. All eyes showed evidence of diabetic retinopathy but to a varying degree. In each case the electroretinogram was recorded on two separate occasions and the results placed in three groups according to the size of the oscillatory potential. The groups were labelled: (a) oscillatory potential absent or barely perceptible; (b) oscillatory potential present but reduced; and (c) oscillatory potential normal. An indication of the distribution of specific retinal lesions within these categories can be seen in Table 9.3. In general the group with an absent oscillatory potential showed more marked fundus changes than the other two groups. Figure 9.3 shows an example of a trace from an early retinopathy; consecutive recordings were made with an interval of about a month between them and the similarity between the two traces is evident. The oscillatory potential was here within normal limits. Figure 9.4 is an example of a trace where the size of the oscillatory potential was reduced and Figure 9.5 is a trace showing absence of the oscillatory potential (Galloway, Wells and Barber, 1972). These figures show the responses from a single intense flash on the light-adapted eye. The early receptor potential is recorded as part of the wave form using this technique, but it did not show any significant changes in this series.

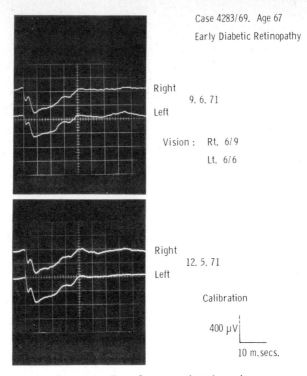

Case 4283/69. Age 67

Early Diabetic Retinopathy

Right
      9. 6. 71
Left

Vision :   Rt. 6/9

            Lt. 6/6

Right
      12. 5. 71
Left

Calibration

400 μV

            10 m.secs.

Figure 9.3.   Trace from an early retinopathy.

Case 697/70. Age 30

Early Diabetic Retinopathy

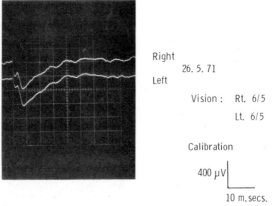

Right
      26. 5. 71
Left

     Vision :   Rt. 6/5

                Lt. 6/5

Calibration

400 μV

            10 m.secs.

Figure 9.4.   Trace with size of oscillatory potential reduced.

Table 9.3. Individual fundus features and the oscillatory potential (OP)

	Absent O.P.	Reduced O.P.	Normal O.P.
Neovascularisation *18 eyes*	14 (78%)	4 (22%)	0
Macula damage *27 eyes*	19 (70%)	5 (19%)	3 (11%)
Venous engorgement *25 eyes*	18 (72%)	3 (12%)	4 (16%)
Hard exudates *24 eyes*	12 (50%)	4 (17%)	8 (33%)
Oedema of post. pole *14 eyes*	12 (86%)	2 (14%)	0

Relationship to the Duration of the Diabetes

In the above series, of the eyes which showed a normal response the average duration of the history of diabetes was 10·1 years, with a range from one year to 24 years. In the case of those eyes which showed an absence of the oscillatory potential, the average duration of the disease was 12·2 years with a range from one year to 29 years.

Relationship to Visual Acuity and Age

In the same series, when the vision was poor the oscillatory potential was nearly always absent, but 12 eyes had good acuity with an absent oscillatory potential. Although it is known that the size of the wavelets becomes less with age, in this particular group of patients the group with absent wavelets showed a slightly younger average age than the normal group. This is presumably a reflection of the severer type of retinopathy which affects the younger age groups.

Case 898/71. Age 54

Diabetic Retinopathy

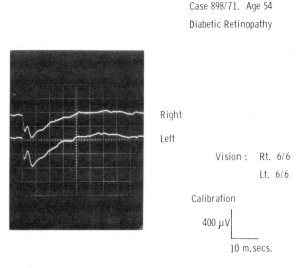

Right

Left

Vision :   Rt. 6/6

Lt. 6/6

Calibration

400 μV

10 m.secs.

Figure 9.5. Trace showing absence of oscillatory potential.

Summary

A selective loss of the oscillatory potential is a feature of diabetic retinopathy and this loss is related to the severe types of retinopathy where the prognosis is often poor. It may also be seen before the appearance of the retinopathy, but it is not clear yet whether this is a bad prognostic sign.

ELECTRODIAGNOSIS IN OCCLUSIVE VASCULAR DISEASE OF THE RETINA

From the early days of clinical electroretinography an interest has been shown in the effect of retinal vascular disease on the electrical response. We have already seen that striking changes can be elicited in patients with diabetic retinopathy and it is now proposed to review the electroretinogram changes which may be seen in other types of vascular disease of the retina.

The retina may be regarded as having a double blood supply, the inner half being supplied by the central retinal artery and the outer half being nourished from the choroidal circulation. Obstruction of the circulation of the central retinal artery might therefore be expected to affect that part of the response which is derived from the inner half of the retina and spare the components of the electroretinogram which originate from the receptors and the pigment epithelium. It will be seen that to some extent this is true. Experiments on monkeys involving selective damage to the choroidal or the retinal circulation have shown that when the *choroidal* circulation is impaired, Granit's PI and PIII components disppear after 20 to 40 minutes. When the retinal circulation is obstructed these components persist for at least an hour. In both instances the 'b' wave disappeard before the PI and the PIII components (Fujino and Hamasaki, 1965). A more striking change which is seen in monkeys when the retinal circulation is clamped is the disappearance of the oscillatory potential and this has considerable clinical significance in man as well as being important evidence for the site of the origin of the wavelets (Brown, 1969) (Figure 9.6).

It has been known for many years that the electroretinogram is highly

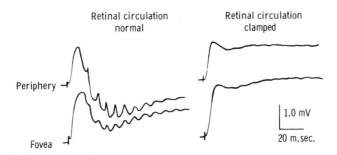

Figure 9.6. Oscillations on the local 'b' waves recorded from the peripheral retina and fovea of cynomolgus monkey and the effect of clamping the retinal circulation. Recording by intraretinal microelectrode. Brown (1969) in 'The Electroretinogram' from *The Retina: Morphology, Function and Clinical Characteristics*, (Ed.) Straatsma, B., Hull, M., Alba, R. A. & Crescitelli, F. *UCLA Forum in Medical Sciences*, No. 8. Originally published by the University of California Press: reprinted by permission of The Regents of the University of California.

sensitive to experimentally induced alterations of blood circulation in the retina and choroid. Experimental methods include pulmonary hyperventilation, hypoxia, aortic compression, and the administration of drugs which affect the systemic blood pressure. Electroretinogram changes in the important vascular diseases of the eye have also been long recognised (Karpe, 1945; Henkes, 1953, 1954ak 1954b; Jayle, Boyer and Saracco, 1965), and they will here be considered in relation to specific vascular lesions.

Occlusion of the Central Retinal Artery

The two characteristic features of the electroretinogram in central artery occlusion are: (1) loss of the oscillatory potential; and (2) a 'negative' type of electroretinogram with enlargement of the 'a' wave and no change or slight diminution of the 'b' wave (Henkes, 1954a; Usami, 1967). Kurimoto et al examined two cases of central retinal artery occlusion with the electroretinogram and fluorescein angiography. Case 1 showed a 'negative' electroretinogram and the angiogram revealed an abnormality of the inferior temporal branch artery and Case 2 showed a diminished 'b' wave and angiography showed extensive disturbance of the retinal circulation. Other reports also indicate that the more severe types of occlusive episode with a poor prognosis show a marked reduction in the size of the 'b' wave whereas the milder types of occlusion may show a 'negative' response. In branch occlusions the electro-

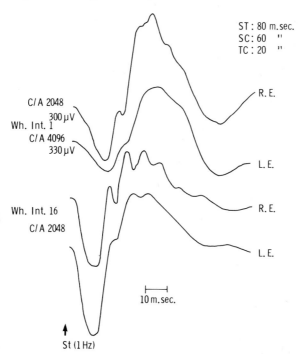

Figure 9.7. Abolition of the wavelets in a case of carotid occlusion on the left side. Reproduced from Stangos et al (1970), *VIIIth ISCERG Symposium.* (Ed.) A. Wirth, Pisa: Pacini, with permission.

retinogram may be normal or minimally affected (Asayama and Takata, 1965; Kurimoto, Watanabe and Kimura, 1968). When the oscillatory potential is examined, a reduction in amplitude or abolition may be seen even in branch artery occlusions. Usami concluded that the wavelets give a good indication of the prognosis in a given case (Usami, 1967).

Ponte examined 19 eyes about one month after the onset of an arterial occlusion involving a branch of the artery only: 52 per cent had a normal electroretinogram (wavelets not examined), 38 per cent had a subnormal response, 8 per cent had a subnormal negative response, and in 2 per cent the response was supernormal. He made the important point that the electro-retinogram may gradually deteriorate over the months following the initial episode (Ponte, 1966). Electroretinogram changes may be delayed, especially in the cases of partial occlusion. The abolition of the wavelets, however, appears to occur shortly after or probably coincidentally with the occlusive episode. Stangos et al examined the oscillatory potential in a wide variety of vascular lesions and showed that, although the reduction in size of the wavelets occurs in many different conditions, it is an almost constant feature of central retinal artery block. All four of their cases of internal carotid insufficiency also showed abnormalities on the affected side. (Stangos et al, 1970) (Figure 9.7). Studies on the acute and late stages of experimental central retinal artery occlusion in the cynomolgus monkey have showed a more subtle change in the ERG. Using a technique of DC recording the authors have shown that very slow oscillations in the amplitude of the 'c' wave were absent, although they are found in normal eyes (Textorius, Skoog and Nilsson, 1978). Studies of the electro-oculogram in occlusion of the central retinal artery show a reduction of the light rise. This finding is a little unexpected; it suggests that the electro-oculogram may not entirely arise in the pigment epithelium and reminds us that our knowledge of the origin of the components of the response is still limited (Nagaya, Hirata and Kaneko, 1970).

Occlusion of the Central Retinal Vein

The findings here are similar to those in central retinal artery occlusion, the commonest change being a subnormal negative response and diminution of the oscillatory potential. The changes are, however, milder than in cases of arterial occlusion. These findings are consistent with Hayreh's observations in monkeys that the typical picture of central retinal vein thrombosis can be produced only when the circulation of both the central retinal artery and vein are blocked (Hayreh, 1965). Arterial insufficiency may be the underlying pathology in both instances, thus explaining the similarity in the electroretinogram changes. In branch retinal vein occlusions the electrical changes are similar to those seen in branch artery occlusions (Ponte, 1966).

Other Vascular Lesions

Henkes detected some electroretinogram differences between patients with arteriosclerosis without arterial hypertension, and patients with hypertension without arteriosclerosis. The former show a subnormal electroretinogram but the latter show a supernormal electroretinogram (Henkes, 1957). Some authors agree with this, others not, and possibly differences arise from the difficulty in defining what is meant by retinal arteriosclerosis (Jayle, Boyer and Saracco, 1965; Vanýsek et al, 1966). According to Ponte, supernormal responses are observed in patients affected by arteriosclerosis with or without general hypertension.

Sometimes patients are referred to the electrodiagnostic clinic with unexplained field defects and systemic hypertension. The electroretinogram can help to decide whether these defects are due to retinal ischaemia or proximal changes in the optic nerve (Thaler, Heilig and Scheiber, 1978).

In five histologically verified cases of temporal arteritis with loss of vision the electroretinogram was normal, indicating ischaemic changes in the optic nerve rather than in the retina. However, many cases of temporal arteritis also show marked retinal arteriosclerotic changes and one would expect to see electroretinogram changes in these patients (Edmund and Jensen, 1967).

The electroretinogram in pulseless disease has been shown to have a reduced 'b' wave and the wavelets were abolished in scotopic conditions (Suyama, 1967). Watanabe and Ando took the opportunity of compressing the carotid artery in a patient with pulseless disease; the 'b' wave became smaller and showed a rebound when the carotid was released. This effect seemed to be specific for pulseless disease (Watanabe and Ando, 1968).

ELECTRODIAGNOSIS IN UVEITIS

Electroretinography has not been widely exploited in uveitis and there is little doubt that its value has been restricted by lack of knowledge on the subject. In general the changes in the trace that might be expected are seen. Thus, in patients with acute iridocyclitis the electroretinogram is quite normal, whereas in patients with chronic iridocyclitis the wavelets and scotopic 'b' waves may be reduced. The electroretinogram may be little affected by central chorioretinitis, but in patients with more extensive posterior uveitis and active disseminated chorioretinitis there may be quite severe impairment of the response (Algvere, 1967). In view of the evidence that the light rise of the electro-oculogram is generated in the pigment epithelium, one might expect earlier changes in this test than with the conventional electroretinogram. This has been shown to be the case (Velissaropoulos, Tsamparlakis and Palimexis, 1968; Wehner, Alexandridis and Bettinger, 1969). Wehner found that the electro-oculogram sometimes showed absence of a light rise in severe cases of disseminated choroiditis.

There is no evidence as yet that the electroretinogram can help us to identify the cause of an attack of uveitis; for example we do not know whether different results are obtained from granulomatous and non-granulomatous types. However, it can indicate the extent or the existence of a fundus lesion and this may sometimes be important clinically. For example, a young patient presented with severe iridocyclitis in an amblyopic eye. As is so often the case, he did not give a clear history of this and at first it was assumed that the failure of his vision to improve was due to involvement of the macular region. Systemic steroids were withheld because of doubt about his previous vision and the mildness of the uveitis; at this point retinoscopy revealed that the affected eye was grossly astigmatic. Although an electroretinogram was not performed in this case, in retrospect it would have been of value in excluding extensive posterior uveitis. In a study of 16 patients suffering from Behçet's disease, the ERGs were examined and compared with those from eleven patients with non-specific posterior uveitis. The amplitude of the 'b' waves was reduced in both cases and found to depend on the extent of the uveitis. In general the rod system was more severely affected than the cone system, and no specific changes were found in the ERG which could distinguish Behçet's disease from the other cases (Hatt and Niemeyer 1976).

Assessment of the extent of fundus involvement becomes extremely important in suspected cases of sympathetic ophthalmitis. Three cases of histologically proven sympathetic ophthalmitis have been examined electroretinographically at varying intervals after the onset of the disease. Initially a 'positive plus' type of response was obtained and this showed a tendency to become 'negative minus' with the passage of time. Similar changes were also seen in the sympathising eye (Georgiades et al, 1966). However, the responses of the electroretinogram following injury must be interpreted with caution. An eye with a perforating wound shows gross electroretinogram changes in the first few days after the injury, and the recovery of the electroretinogram after injury has yet to be accurately assessed in a variety of cases. Here then we have another situation where the value of the test is limited by our lack of knowledge.

Animal experiments can throw some light on the relationship of the response to the disease process. For example, Algvere injected horse serum into the vitreous of a series of sensitised pigeons. The 'a' wave showed a progressive reduction in amplitude with repeated injections as well as the oscillatory potential. Histologically it was shown that the oscillatory wavelets were affected in those pigeons with diffuse involvement of the retina, whereas when the 'a' wave was mainly involved, the damage tended to be limited to the receptors (Algvere, Hediw and Kock, 1968).

Patients who have suffered disseminated choroiditis in the past may present with scattered pigmentation in the fundus, and the presence of a normal or subnormal electroretinogram can help to distinguish these patients from those suffering from retinitis pigmentosa (Figure 9.8).

CHOROIDITIS

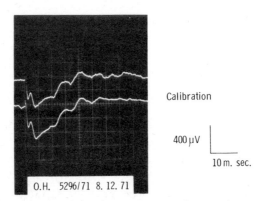

Calibration

400 µV

10 m. sec.

O.H.   5296/71 8. 12. 71

Figure 9.8. Response from a patient with healed disseminated choroiditis of unknown aetiology. The fundus showed scattered pigmentation.

Electrodiagnostic tests in uveitis have not therefore been exploited to the full and there would appear to be a place for routine testing of cases where the extent of choroidal involvement is difficult to assess by other means. There may also be a place for the electroretinogram in assessing the state of the eye prior to cataract surgery in cases of chronic uveitis, and in particular an electroretinogram is indicated in suspected sympathetic ophthalmitis.

ELECTRODIAGNOSIS IN DISEASES OF THE OPTIC NERVE

For many years it has been generally accepted and confirmed by animal work that damage to the optic nerve does not affect the electrical response from the retina. Histological evidence also confirms this in that the part of the retina which is thought to give rise to the response is not damaged in patients with optic atrophy. This fact provides a serious pitfall in the interpretation of electroretinogram traces; an eye may be completely blind from glaucoma and yet show a normal electroretinogram. In fact minor changes in the photopic components of the electroretinogram have been described in chronic glaucoma, but these are slight (Alvis, 1966; Ogata, 1976). The visually evoked response may well prove to be an important supplementary test in these cases. It has been shown that in cases of traumatic optic atrophy, the visually evoked response showed changes in proportion to the amount of visual loss whereas the electroretinogram remained normal (Plane et al, 1969). The electroretinogram has also been reported as normal in patients with congenital unilateral hypoplasia of the optic nerve (Ewald, 1967; Francois and de Rouck, 1976), but in a family suffering from dominant juvenile optic atrophy the photopic electroretinogram was affected and the flicker fusion frequency was also lower than normal (Hellner and Haase, 1967). The fact that some patients with optic nerve atrophy seem to have a supernormal response has excited some interest and there are several authentic reports of the phenomenon (Samson, Samson and Tanay, 1966; Auerbach, 1966; Gills, 1966). It has been suggested that the increase in amplitude of the electroretinogram may be due to the division of centrifugal fibres in the optic nerve; these fibres may normally have an inhibitory influence on the size of the response. Some interesting evidence of the value of this form of test is seen in two patients suffering from optic nerve compression by a tuberculum sellae meningioma (Feinsod and Auerbach, 1971). The damage to the optic nerve could be demonstrated by the reduced or absent visually evoked response. In one case the amplitudes of the electroretinogram were enhanced. After the tumour had been removed, the visually evoked response improved as the visual acuity improved. In both patients decompression was accompanied by a decrease in amplitude of the electroretinogram (see also Ikeda, Tremain and Sanders, 1978).

In general, any changes that are seen in the electroretinogram appear to be minimal and the visually evoked response provides a more valid clinical test.

The VEP in retrobulbar neuritis

A high incidence of abnormal patterned VEPs in patients suffering from retrobulbar neuritis was described by Halliday et al (1972); this in itself would not have been of clinical interest were it not for the fact that more subtle changes in the VEP could be seen to persist long after the clinical signs of optic neuritis had subsided. A test of previously healed optic neuritis is of more value to the clinician than a test of active disease, which is already detectable by routine clinical methods. Therefore it was of special interest when Halliday and several others showed that the latency of the major peaks in the transient VEP to pattern reversal is increased and may remain increased for several years following an acute attack. This delay in the response is best shown by comparing the response from the two eyes. During an acute attack of retrobulbar neuritis, when the visual acuity is severely impaired, the VEP is severely affected. In some cases the response from the affected eye is abolished altogether. As the vision recovers, the amplitude of the VEP returns towards its normal value, but a characteristic slight delay in the response remains. It has also been shown that a surprisingly large number of supposedly normal eyes in patients with multiple sclerosis give abnormal results when the VEP is checked. This delay in the response is not of course specifically seen in demyelinating disease; other possible causes of an altered response such as amblyopia or macular disease must be excluded. Other evoked responses have also been investigated in multiple sclerosis and a measuring of a variety of evoked responses can provide diagnostic evidence in suspected cases (Mastaglia et al, 1976, Wilberger, 1976, Paty et al, 1976, Asselman et al, 1975). The VEP recorded from a patient with acute retrobulbar neuritis is shown in Fig. 9.9. It can be seen that the response from the right side is greatly impaired.

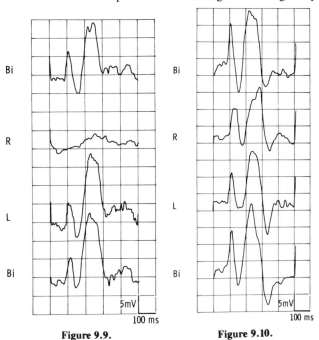

Figure 9.9.   **Figure 9.10.**

Figure 9.9. VEP in a patient suffering from an acute attack of retrobulbar neuritis in the right eye. Note the markedly reduced amplitude on the right side.

Figure 9.10. VEP in the same patient as in Figure 9.9 after he had recovered from an attack of retrobulbar neuritis in the right eye. Note that the first negative peak in particular is very slightly delayed compared with the left. The difference is small but significant.

The VEP recorded from the same patient four months later is shown in Fig. 9.10. Although the response from the right eye has apparently recovered, careful inspection shows a delay in the latency of all the major components. It is this slight change that enables the electrodiagnostician to say whether a patient has suffered from retrobulbar neuritis in the past, and the change may persist after other clinical evidence of the attack has disappeared.

The VEP in tobacco amblyopia

The amplitude of the VEP is sensitive to changes in visual acuity, as has already been shown, during an acute attack of optic neuritis, where the response may be abolished altogether. Similar findings have been recorded in patients with tobacco amblyopia where it is possible to monitor the recovery by measuring the VEP at intervals when the patient has abstained from tobacco. In some of these patients the normal positive peak at about 100 msec may be inverted (Halliday 1976; Fig. 9.11).

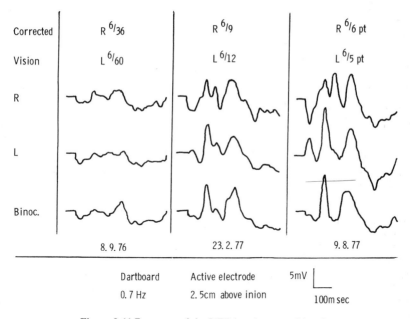

Figure 9.11 Recovery of the VEP in tobacco amblyopia.

The VEP in chronic glaucoma

Already quite successful attempts have been made to relate VEP changes to visual field defects. A purely objective test for field changes in glaucoma could prove very useful when the question of glaucoma surgery may depend on an increase in field loss. Clear-cut alterations in phase and amplitude have been demonstrated in patients with glaucomatous field defects. This was achieved by examining steady-state visually evoked responses to pattern reversal stimulation of retinal areas corresponding to discrete field quadrants (Cappin and Nissim, 1975; Fig. 9.12).

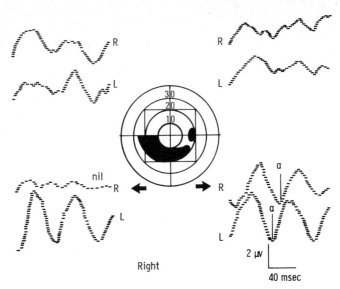

Figure 9.12 The VEP in a patient with a glaucomatous field defect in the right eye. The stimulus was applied to different quadrants of the central field using midline electrodes. Note the diminished response on stimulating the lower nasal quadrant of the right eye (Cappin and Nissim, 1975).

The VEP and other diseases of the optic nerve

The VEP has been measured in Tay-Sachs disease: an absent VEP and a normal ERG is the usual finding. This is the result that one might expect from a lesion at the level of the retinal ganglion cells, which involved central vision (Honda and Sudo, 1976).

It is possible to monitor the function of the optic nerve by means of the VEP and this technique has been practised in orbital surgery. Permanent loss of vision following surgery is a recognised risk, particularly when hypotensive anaesthesia is being used. Wright et al have described a method of monitoring the function of the optic nerve which entails continuously stimulating the retina with an unstructured stimulus and recording the VEP throughout the operation (Wright et al, 1973).

It can be seen then that a knowledge of the electrodiagnostic changes in diseases of the optic nerve is essential when interpreting these responses in general. A surgeon who is encouraged to remove a cataract on the grounds of a normal electroretinogram alone may be unpleasantly surprised at the poor visual result if he been led astray by an inadequate electrodiagnostic report.

ELECTRODIAGNOSIS WHEN THE FUNDUS IS NORMAL

It has already been shown in the previous chapter that the optic fundus may be normal in the early stages of retinitis pigmentosa, and in these instances the value of the electroretinogram is well proven. It has also been shown that the VEP is markedly altered in acute retrobulbar neuritis, and although in such cases the pupil reaction is impaired on the affected side, the VEP can provide helpful supporting evidence of an organic lesion in the visual pathway. There are several other instances when the patient may present with unilateral deterioration of vision and yet on examination be found to have a normal fundus. These will now be discussed.

Amblyopia of Disuse

The reduction of visual acuity that can be seen in association with squint or anisometropia with no visible abnormality in the retina would seem to be an ideal subject for VEP studies, especially if we assume that the VEP arises in the primary visual cortex. VEP studies might be expected to tell us something about the site of the defect in this group of ambylopias. In general the pattern VEP recorded by stimulating the affected eye shows a reduction in amplitude; this is in contrast to the electroretinogram as routinely recorded and the flash VEP, which are usually quite normal (Tsutsui et al, 1973; Arden et al, 1974). It is not at present possible to distinguish between the different types of amblyopia of disuse using the VEP, but some interesting facts are emerging. For example a 'binocular negative' effect has been described in which the binocular VEP is smaller than the VEP recorded from each eye individually. In normal subjects the binocular VEP is larger than the response from the individual eyes and can be seen to represent the sum of the waveform of the two. This binocular negative effect would appear to represent some form of suppression and it is found more frequently in strabismic amblyopia (Tsutsui et al, 1973). Attempts to correlate the VEP with some of the psychophysical findings in amblyopia seem to indicate defects both peripheral to and beyond the primary visual cortex (Lawwill et al, 1973). In the normal eye the VEP shows a maximum amplitude with fifteen-minute checks, the response is smaller when the stimulus is composed of either larger or smaller checks. In one careful study of an adult amblyope, the affected eye showed a maximum amplitude at the sixty-minute check size. In addition to a shift in the peak amplitude for the amblyopic eye there was a significantly larger signal for the sixty-minute check from the amblyopic eye than from the normal eye. Furthermore, when a small-field three-degree stimulus was used there was no difference in amplitude between the normal and amblyopic eye. It has been suggested that in the amblyope, the normal central three-degree area is unable to exert sufficient lateral inhibitory effect on the surrounding retina and it has been further suggested that the well-recognised increase in visual acuity with separate letter testing which is found with some amblyopes may be due to the fact that they are looking at each letter in a manner equivalent to a small-field pattern stimulus (Sokol, 1977).

A different light has been thrown on the study of this type of amblyopia by the examination of subjects with high degrees of astigmatism. It is known that the resolving power of the human visual system is better in the vertical and horizontal orientation than the two oblique orientations. The same effect can be seen in the VEP (Campbell and Maffei, 1970). When astigmatic subjects are examined, a high proportion show a reduction in the amplitude of the VEP when a grating stimulus is orientated in the meridian with the lower refractive error. This impairment of the VEP occurs even with full spectacle correction. (Fiorentini and Maffei, 1973; Freeman and Thibos, 1973; Maffei, 1977).

Hemianopia

Sometimes the ophthalmic surgeon may be puzzled by an apparent reduction in visual acuity and subsequently find that it is due to a homonymous hemianopia. In the very young and the very old these defects may not be easy to pick up, so it is of special interest to consider some of the recently described VEP findings. The use of an unstructured flash stimulus together with laterally placed electrodes can give asymmetrical responses from the two sides in hemianopic patients, but by and large such results have not proved very reliable. The use of a patterned hemifield stimulus seems to be more promising. Blumhardt et al have shown that a hemifield pattern-reversal stimulus produces a

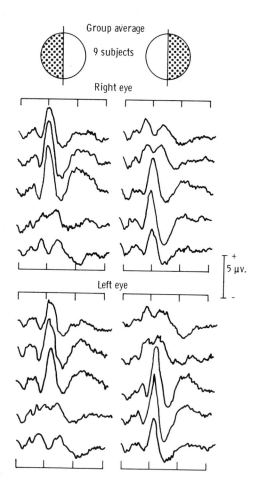

Figure 9.13 Group average of monocular responses from nine healthy subjects. Stimulated halffields shown checkered. Traces from top to bottom in each instance represent recordings from a transverse chain of electrodes placed symmetrically at 5-cm intervals across the scalp from left to right. Pattern reversal. Note the larger response over the ipsilateral hemisphere (Blumhardt, Barrett and Halliday, 1977).

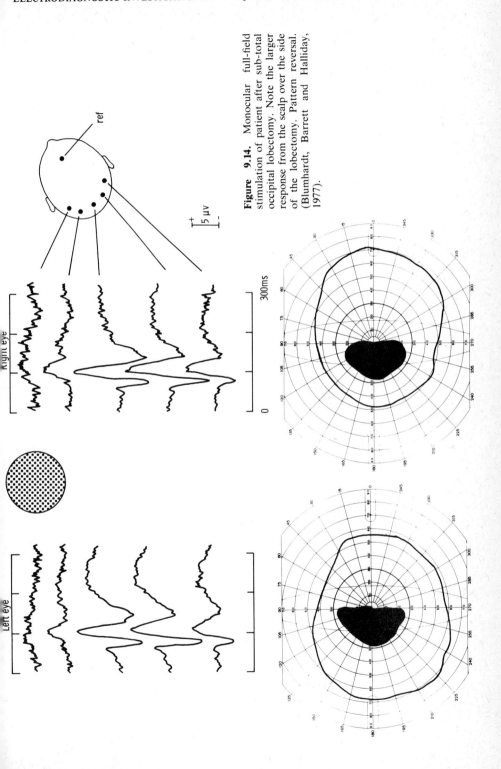

Figure 9.14. Monocular full-field stimulation of patient after sub-total occipital lobectomy. Note the larger response from the scalp over the side of the lobectomy. Pattern reversal. (Blumhardt, Barrett and Halliday, 1977).

larger response from the electrodes placed over the ipsilateral hemisphere than over the contralateral hemisphere. These investigators stress the use of pattern reversal every 600 msec and the placing of electrodes in a transverse chain of five, five cm above the inion and five cm apart, the indifferent electrode being placed on the forehead. This system produces the type of paradoxical response already described in Chapter 4, the smaller contralateral response is usually out of phase with the ipsilateral one. A full-field pattern stimulus tends to produce the summed effect of the two half-field responses. Because the responses from each half-field are out of phase when recorded through a single laterally placed electrode, the sum of the responses may be zero or, at most, very small. This means that full-field stimulation gives a large midline response but smaller or absent responses from laterally placed electrodes (Blumhardt, Barrett and Halliday, 1977).

Full-field and hemifield stimulation of patients with homonymous and bitemporal hemianopias gives predictable results using this technique (Figs. 9.13 and 9.14). (Blumhardt et al, 1977). The exact position of the electrodes and the specifications of the stimulus appear to be important, because other workers obtained what at first appeared to be conflicting results (Wildberger, Van Lith and Wijngaarde, 1976).

The rather surprising finding that a larger response is found over the inert hemisphere has been confirmed in a patient who had undergone an occipital lobectomy, which suggests that the electrical changes must be projected from the active side directly to the scalp rather than through the corpus callosum (Fig. 9.14).

Hysterical Blindness

True hysterical blindness is extremely rare and presumably the VEP would be normal in these patients. Unfortunately, difficulties arise in that some normal subjects have very small VEPs. It is also possible for the hysteric to give a misleading result by not fixing on the stimulus. In my own clinical experience hysterics and malingerers often fail to keep their appointment for the electro-diagnostic clinic.

SUMMARY

The abundance of research literature on the subject of electrodiagnosis is an indication that much still remains to be learned about its clinical application. In this chapter we have seen that definite information can be obtained in a variety of acquired diseases of the retina and optic nerve. It is important that electrodiagnosis is reserved for the most suitable cases and that the recordings are interpreted by a clinician before being recorded in the notes.

REFERENCES

Algvere, P. (1967) Electroretinographic studies on posterior uveitis. *Acta Ophthalmologica*, **45**, 299–313.
Algvere, P., Hediw, A. & Kock, E. (1968) The electroretinogram and histopathology in experimental uveitis of the pigeon. *Acta Ophthalmologica*, **46**, 920–935.
Alvis, D. L. (1966) Electroretinographic changes in controlled open angle glaucoma. *American Journal of Ophthalmology*, **61**, 121–131.

Asayama, R., Nagata, M., Konno, S. & Shibata, A. (1957) Electroretinography in retinal detachment. *Japanese Journal of Clinical Ophthalmology*, **11**, 304–321.

Asayama, R. & Takata, H. (1965) Occlusion of central retinal artery and electroretinogram. *Acta societatis Ophthalmologicae Japonicae*, **68**, 155–161.

Asselman, P., Chadwick, D. W. & Marsden, C. (1975) Visual evoked responses in diagnosis and management of patients suspected of multiple sclerosis. *Brain*, **98**, 261.

Auerbach, E. (1966) In discussion on 'Electroretinograms in some diseases of the optic pathways'. *Vth ISCERG Symposium (Ghent)*, pp. 25–31. In *The Clinical Value of Electroretinography*. Basel/New York: Karger.

Blach, R. K. & Behrman, J. (1967) The electrical activity of the eye in retinal detachment. *Transactions of the Ophthalmological Society of the United Kingdom*, **87**, 263–266.

Blumhardt, L. C., Barrett, G. & Halliday, A. M. (1977) The asymmetrical VER to pattern reversal in one half field and its significance for analysis of field defects. *British Journal of Ophthalmology*, **61**, 454.

Brown, K. T. (1969) The electroretinogram. In *The Retina: Morphology, Function and Clinical Characteristics*, p. 363. (Ed.) Straatsma, B., Hull, M., Alba, R. A. & Crescitelli, F. University of California Forum for Medical Science: University of California Press.

Campbell, F. W. & Maffei, L. (1970) Electrophysiological evidence for the existence of orientation and size detectors in the human visual system. *Journal of Physiology* (London), **207**, 635.

Cappin, J. & Nissim, S. (1975) VER in assessment of field defects in glaucoma. *Archives of Ophthalmology*, **93** 9.

Edmund, J. & Jensen, S. (1967) The electroretinogram in temporal arteritis. *Acta Ophthalmologica*, **45**, 601–609.

Ewald, R. A. (1967) Three cases of unilateral hypoplasia of the optic nerve. *American Journal of Ophthalmology*, **63**, 763–767.

Feinsod, M. & Auerbach, E. (1971) The electroretinogram and the visual evoked potential in two patients with tuberculum sellae meningioma, before and after decompression of the optic nerve. *Ophthalmologica*, **163**, 360–368.

Fiorentini, A. & Maffei, L. (1973) Evoked potentials in astigmatic subjects. *Vision Research*, **13**, 1781.

Francois, J. & De Rouck, A. (1955) L'électrorétinographie dans la myopie et les décollements myopigenes de la rétine. *Acta Ophthalmologica*, **33**, 131–155.

Francois, J. & De Rouck, A. (1976) Electroretinographic study of hypoplasia of the optic nerve. *Ophthalmologica* (Basel), **172**, 308–330.

Freeman, R. E. & Thibos, L. N. (1973) Electrophysiological evidence that abnormal early visual experience can modify the human brain. *Science* (New York), **180**, 876–8.

Fujino, T. & Hamasaki, D. (1965) The effect of occluding the retinal and choroidal circulations on the electroretinogram of monkeys. *Journal of Physiology*, **180**, 837–845.

Galloway, N. R. (1970) Degeneration of receptors and the early receptor potential. *Proceedings of the VIIIth ISCERG Symposium*, p. 154. (Ed.) Wirth, Alberto. Pisa: Pacini.

Galloway, N. R., Wells, M. & Barber, C. (1972) Changes in the oscillatory potential in relation to different features of diabetic retinopathy. *IXth Symposium of ISCERG (Brighton)*. In *The Visual System*, p. 275. (ED.) Arden, G. B. London: Plenum.

Georgiades, G., Paltakis, P., Stangos, N. & Castanas, D. (1966) A study of the electroretinographic signs in four cases of sympathetic ophthalmitis. *Archives of the Ophthalmological Society of Northern Greece*, **15**, 6–18.

Gills, J. P. (1966) The electroretinogram after section of the optic nerve in man. *American Journal of Ophthalmology*, **62**, 287–291.

Halliday, A. M. (1976) Visually evoked response in optic nerve disease. *Transactions of the Ophthalmological Society of the United Kingdom*, **96**, 372.

Hatt, M. & Niemeyer, G. (1976) The ERG in Behcet's disease. *Albrecht von Graefes Archiv für klinische und experimentelle Ophthalmologie*, **198**, 112–120.

Hayreh, S. S. (1965) Occlusion of the central retinal vessels. *British Journal of Ophthalmology*, **49**, 626–645.

Hellner, K. A. & Haase, W. (1967) Electroretinographic findings in dominant juvenile optic atrophy. *Albrecht von Graefes Archiv für Ophthalmologie*, **172**, 152–163.

Henkes, H. E. (1953) Electroretinography in circulatory disturbances of the retina (I). Electroretinogram in cases of occlusion of central retinal vein or one of its branches. *American Medical Association: Archives of Ophthalmology*, **49**, 190–201.

Henkes, H. E. (1954a) electroretinography in circulatory disturbances of the retina (II). The electroretinogram in cases of occlusion of central retinal artery or one of its branches. *Archives of Ophthalmology*, **51**, 42–53.

Henkes, H. E. (1954b) Electroretinography in circulatory disturbances of the retina (IV). Electroretinogram in cases of retinal and choroidal hypertension and arteriosclerosis. *American Medical Association: Archives of Ophthalmology*, **52**, 30–41.

Henkes, H. E. (1957) Electroretinography. An evaluation of the influence of retinal and general metabolic conditions on the electrical response of the retina. *American Journal of Ophthalmology*, **43**, 67–81.

Honda, Y. & Sudo, M. (1976) Electroretinogram and visually evoked cortical potential in Tay Sachs disease. Report of two cases. *Journal of Pediatric Ophthalmology*, **13**, 226.

Ikeda, H., Tremain, K. E. & Sanders, M. D. (1978) Neurophysiological investigation in optic nerve disease: combined assessment of the visual evoked response and electroretinogram. *British Journal of Ophthalmology* (London), **62**, 227–239.

Jacobson, J. H., Basar, D., Carrol, J., Stephens, G. & Saphir, A. (1958) The electroretinogram as a prognostic aid in retinal detachment. *American Medical Association: Archives of Ophthalmology*, **59**, 515–520.

Jaÿle, G–E., Boyer, R. L. & Saracco, J. B. (1965) *L'électrorétinographie. Bases Physiologiques et Données Cliniques*. Paris: Masson.

Karpe, G. (1945) The basis of clinical electoretinography. *Acta Ophthalmologica*, **24**, 118.

Karpe, G. (1948) The electroretinogram in detachment of the retina. *Acta Ophthalmologica*, **26**, 267.

Kurachi, Y., Yonemura, D., Hatta, M., Tsuchida, Y. & Yamada, Y. (1966) Oscillatory potential in diabetic retinopathy. *Folia Ophthalmologica Japonica*, **17**, 375–378.

Kurimoto, B., Watanbe, T. & Kimura. (1968) Electroretinographical and fluorographical studies on occlusion of the central retinal artery. *Folia Ophthalmologica Japonica*, **21**, 197–202.

Lawwill, T., Cox, W. E., Tuttle, D., Meur, G. & Burian, H. (1973) Lateral inhibition and the VER in central field of an amblyope. *Investigative Ophthalmology*, **12**, 154.

Lobes, L. A. (1978) The electro-oculogram in human retinal detachment. *British Journal of Ophthalmology*, **62**, 223.

Maffei, L. (1977) Visual potentials evoked by gratings in normal and astigmatic subjects. In: *Visual Evoked Potentials in Man: New Developments*. Ed. J. E. Desmedt. pp. 395–400. Oxford: Clarendon Press.

Mastaglia, F. L., Black, J. L. & Collins, D. W. K. (1976) Evoked potential studies in neurological disorders. *Proceedings of the Australian Association of Neurologists*, **13**, 15–23.

Nagaya, T., Hirata, A. & Kaneko, T. (1970) Electrophysiological studies on occlusion of central retinal artery. *Folia Ophthalmologica Japonica*, **21**, 197–202.

Ogata, W. (1976) Electrophysiological study on glaucoma. I. The electroretinogram in primary glaucoma. *Acta. Societas Ophthalmologica Japonica*, **80**, 1555–1564.

Parizot, H. (1967) L'électrorétinographie et le pronostic des interventions chirurgicales pour décollement de rétine. *Bulletin des Sociétés d'Ophthalmologie de France*, **67**, 434–444.

Paty, J., Brendt, P. L., Henry, P. & Faure, J. M. A. (1976) Potentials evoqués visuels et sclerose en plaques (1) *Revue Neurologique*, **132**, 9, 605.

Plane, C., Sole, P., Janny, P., Montrieul, B. & Rouber, F. (1969) The value of electrophysiological examination of the optic nerve cut by orbital trauma. *Rivista Oto-Neuro-Oftalmologica*, **41**, 73–83.

Ponte, F. (1966) Electroretinogram and vascular disturbance. The clinical value of electroretinography. *Vth Symposium of ISCERG (Ghent)*, pp. 300–311. Basel/New York: Karger. (Published 1968).

Rendahl, I. (1961) The clinical electroretinogram in detachment of the retina. *Acta Ophthalmologica*, **64**, 1–83.

Samson-Dollfus, D., Samson, M. & Tanay, A. (1966) Electroretinograms in some diseases of the optic pathways. *Vth Symposium of ISCERG (Ghent)*, pp. 25–31. In *The Clinical Value of Electroretinography*. Basel/New York: Karger.

Schmöger, E. (1957) Die prognostische Bedentung des Elektroretinogramms bei Ablatio retinae. *Klinische Monatsblätter für Augenheilkunde*, **131**, 335–343.

Scott, G. I. (1953) Ocular complications of diabetes mellitus. *British Journal of Ophthalmology*, **37**, 705–715.

Simonsen, S. E. (1966) Electroretinogram in diabetics. *Vth Symposium of ISCERG (Ghent)*. In *The Clinical Value of Electroretinography*, pp. 403–412. Basel/New York: Karger.

Sokol, S. (1977) Visual evoked potentials to checkerboard pattern stimuli in strabismic amblyopia. In: *Visual Evoked Potentials in Man: New Developments*. Ed. J. E. Desmedt. Pp. 410–417 Oxford: Clarendon Press.

Stangos, N., Rey, P., Meyer, J. & Thorens, B. (1970) Averaged electroretinogram responses in normal human subjects and ophthalmological patients. *VIIIth Symposium of ISCERG, pp. 277–304. (Ed.) Wirth, Alberto. Pisa: Pacini.*

Sundmark, E. (1958) The electroretinogram and malignant intraocular tumours. *Acta Ophthalmologica*, **36**, 57–64.

Suyama, T. (1967) A case of pulseless disease. *Folia Ophthalmologica Japonica*, **18**, 1100–1105.

Tamai, A. (1977) Electrophysiological studies on the fellow eyes (so-called healthy eyes) of patients with idiopathic retina. II Scotopic ERG findings. *Folia Ophthalmologica Japonica*, **28**, 816–819.

Tamai, A. (1978) Studies on the ERP in the human eye. ERP in the fellow eyes of patients with idiopathic retinal detachment. *Documenta Ophthalmologica* (Proceedings Series), **15**, 279.

Tassy, A., Jayle, G–E. & Gastaut-Maysou, M. (1971) Eléctrorétinographie classique et potentiel oscillatoire dans le diabète et dans la cataracte du sujet diabètique. *Archives d'Ophthalmologie*, **31**, 413–426.

Textorius, O., Skoog, K. O. & Nilsson, S. E. G. (1978) Studies on acute and late stages of experimental central retinal artery occlusion in the cynomolgus monkey. II. Influence on the cyclic changes in the amplitude of the 'c' wave of the ERG and in the standing potential of the eye. *Acta Ophthalmologica*, **56**, 665–676.

Thaler, A., Heilig, P. & Scheiber, V. (1978) The ERG off-response in ischaemic retinopathy. *Ophthalmic Research*, **10**, 237.

Tsutsui, J., Nakamura, Y., Takenaka, J. & Fukai, S. (1973) Abnormalities of VER in types of amblyopia. *Japanese Journal of Clinical Ophthalmology*, **17**, 83.

Usami, E. (1967) The electroretinogram in occlusion of the retinal vessels. *Acta Societatis Ophthalmologicae Japonicae*, **71**, 39–45.

Vanýsek, J., Hrachovina, V., Anton, M. & Moster, M. (1966) The electroretinogram in some circulatory and metabolic disorders. *Vth ISCERG Symposium (Ghent)*, held in conjunction with the *XXth International Congress of Ophthalmology*, Munich. In *The Clinical Value of Electroretinography* (Ed.) Francois, J. pp. 312–330. Basel/New York: Karger. (Published 1968).

Velissaropoulos, P., Tsamparlakis, J. & Palimexis, G. (1968) A comparative study of electro-oculogram and electroretinogram in some ocular diseases. *Bulletin de la Société Hellénique d'Ophthalmologie*, **36**, 58–76.

Watanabe, I. & Ando, F. (1968) The effect of carotid artery compression on the electroretinogram. *Acta Societatis Ophthalmologicae Japonicae*, **72**, 822–828.

Wehner, F., Alexandridis, E. & Bettinger, F. (1969) Changes of potential of electro-oculogram compared with normal eyes and after healing. *Bericht deutsche ophthalmologische Gesellschaft*, **70**, 161–165.

Wildberger, H. (1976) Retrobulbar neuritis and visual evoked cortical potentials. *Klinische Monatsblätter für Augenheilkunde*, **168**, 88–100.

Wildberger, H., Van Lith, G. W., Wijngaarde, R. (1976) VECP in evaluation of homonymous and bitemporal field defects. *British Journal of Ophthalmology*, **60**, 273.

Yonemura, D., Aoki, T. & Tsuzuki, K. (1962) Electroretinogram in diabetic retinopathy. *Archives of Ophthalmology*, **68**, 19–24.

Yonemura, D., Kawasaki, K., Kawasaki, C. & Usukura, H. (1972b) The oscillatory potential of the electroretinogram in idiopathic detachment of the retina. *Acta Societatis Ophthalmologicae Japonicae*, **76**, 267–270.

Yonemura, D., Kawasaki, K., Kunita, M. & Ron, K. (1972a) A statistical study of the oscillatory potential of the electroretinogram in diabetes mellitus. *Folia Ophthalmologica Japonica*, **23**, 93–96.

CHAPTER TEN

The Effect of Opacities in the Media on the Response

From the early days of clinical electroretinography is has been apparent that opacities in the media have remarkably little effect on the retinal response. Much of the clinical value of electroretinography relies on this fact, and it is therefore perhaps surprising that the exact manner in which light is transmitted by opaque media has not been extensively studied. The manner in which the recorded electrical changes may be influenced by different types of opacity has also received little attention. On the other hand, every electroretinographer is familiar with the fact that a normal response may be recorded through extremely dense opacities. As far as we know, the site of the opacity, that is to say whether it is in the cornea or posterior to it, does not make any difference to its diffusing or filtering effect.

Quite frequently it is necessary to perform surgery on an eye with opaque media and the clinician relies on evidence from tests of light perception and light projection. In some cases, due to senility, low intelligence or language difficulties these tests may not be reliable and the electroretinogram can be very useful here.

It is convenient to consider these opacities as: (1) corneal; (2) in the anterior chamber; (3) in the lens; and (4) in the vitreous. One might include here the possibility of an electrodiagnostic investigation with the eyes closed. Occasionally, following contusion injuries of the orbit, massive swelling of the eyelids can prevent an examination of the fundus; it is possible to obtain an electroretinogram and an electro-oculogram through the closed lids with a strong stimulus, although under these circumstances a wick electrode would have to be used rather than a contact lens. So far as I am aware this technique has never been put into practice, although the electro-oculogram has been used in a rather different way to measure eye movements in sleep.

CORNEAL OPACITIES

Now that special units for corneal grafting and for the insertion of corneal prostheses are being formed, it seems possible that a place will be found for routine pre-operative electrodiagnostic investigations. It may be necessary to assess retinal function prior to tattooing an unsightly corneal scar, for example, but there are numerous other instances where an electroretinogram can help and two cases are described here to illustrate this:

CASE 1. No. 1162/69. Female aged 25. This patient developed Stevens-Johnson syndrome after suffering a urinary infection which had been treated by sulphonamides. The skin changes were extremely severe so that the patient's life was in jeopardy at one point. The eye changes were also very severe with recurrent corneal ulceration and superimposed infection with *Pseudomonas pyocyanea*. As the condition became less active, examination of the eyes showed bilateral corneal scarring and shrinkage of the conjunctiva. Three corneal grafts have left the patient with sufficient vision to be reasonably independent and an electroretinogram was performed before the final corneal grafting operation. The result of this can be seen in Figure 10.1. The trace is not normal; the 'a' wave has a rounded peak and the wavelets on the 'b' wave are absent. The early receptor potential is also very small. Some of these changes could be due to the opaque media but there would appear to be ischaemic changes in the retina of some kind. Since the cornea is still not clear it has not been possible to confirm this by fundus examination. However, in this case the amplitude of the electroretinogram was sufficiently great to make us feel that a further graft was justified.

Case No. 1162/69

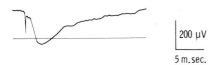

200 µV

5 m.sec.

Figure 10.1. Electroretinogram from a case of Stevens-Johnson disease with dense corneal opacity.

CASE 2. No. 4943/71. Male aged eight. This boy suffered a contusion injury of the right eye which produced a full hyphaema followed by intractable secondary glaucoma. The anterior chamber was washed out, but further bleeding occurred and the recurrence of secondary glaucoma was barely controlled by Diamox. The patient was left with a recurrently irritable eye with an opaque white cornea. Light projection was fair but in view of the persistent irritation the eye was enucleated about one year after the injury. The enucleation was performed in spite of a relatively normal electroretinogram (Figure 10.2). The trace is normal apart from absence of the early receptor potential and this may be due to the opacity of the cornea. Histological examination of the eye showed that the retina was healthy, the disc was not cupped and there was no evidence of sympathetic ophthalmitis. There were several reasons why the result of the electroretinogram was ignored; the parents were very concerned about the possibility of involvement of the other eye, and a second opinion advised enucleation. Had we performed a visually evoked response here and demonstrated a response a different decision might have been justified.

Case No. 4943/71

Figure 10.2. Electroretinogram from a patient with an opaque cornea following trauma.

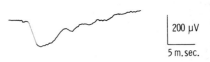

200 µV

5 m.sec.

Opacities in the Anterior Chamber

Acute iridocyclitis does not usually produce electroretinogram changes, but an electroretinogram is sometimes a useful test in these patients when a degree of associated choroiditis is also suspected. This applies particularly following perforated wounds in children when sympathetic ophthalmitis may be suspected. In this kind of situation where the electroretinogram may offer some extra information without greatly influencing the line of treatment, the value of the test would be greatly enhanced if it was readily available. Unfortunately the equipment is still relatively cumbersome, too bulky to fit on the consultant's desk in fact, and by its geographical position in the hospital its use must be reserved for the more difficult diagnostic problems. From the point of view of research, however, it is useful to investigate these cases; for example we do not know the exact attenuating effect of blood in the anterior chamber which limits our ability to interpret from patients with traumatic hyphaema.

Opacities in the Lens

As might be expected, most of the work on opaque media has concerned cataracts. Recent investigation of 20 eyes with mature cataracts showed that 16 had normal pre-operative electroretinograms and the post-operative visual acuity of these ranged between 6/12 and 6/6. In three cases the 'b' wave was reduced pre-operatively and the post-operative vision was limited to about 3/36. In one case a markedly diminished 'b' wave was recorded and after surgery fundus examination revealed scarring from chorioretinitis and the vision was less than 6/60 (Tsinopoulos, Karyophyllis and Konstas, 1972). In another more detailed investigation of 68 eyes some interesting findings were noted; in this series, of the eyes with normal pre-operative electroretinograms, 92 per cent had a postoperative visual acuity of 6/6 or better. In the case of those eyes with abnormal pre-operative electroretinograms only 22 per cent had a visual acuity of 6/6 after the operation. Apart from conventional electroretinography these patients were also tested with a red stimulus subtending 3° at the eye, and using this stimulus the 'b' wave was rather larger in the cataractous eyes than in the aphakic eyes (Mikawa and Tamura, 1970). This somewhat unexpected finding has been also described by Burian and Burns (1966); they recorded electroretinograms pre- and post-operatively in 37 eyes of 22 patients with senile cataracts with ages ranging from 59 to 88 years. They used stimuli of different intensity levels and showed that in 23 eyes the 'b' wave amplitude was generally lower in the aphakic state. In five eyes the 'b' wave amplitude was higher in the aphakic state and in another five there was no difference pre- and post-operatively. This decrease in the size of the response after the cataract had been removed was more evident at lower stimulus intensities (Figure 10.3). In eyes with mature cataracts this effect was less evident and in fact in those cases the post-operative response tended to be slightly larger. Burian and Burns claimed that the cataractous lens acts as a diffusing screen in some cases and this could explain how the effect of low intensity stimuli is particularly enhanced. With flashes of high intensity the rods are saturated in both the phakic and the aphakic state, and under these

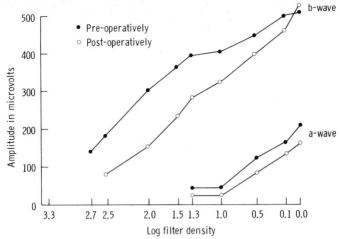

Figure 10.3. Pre- and post-operative amplitudes of 'a' and 'b' waves on a single patient at ten different intensities of white light. Reproduced from Burian, H. M. & Burns, C. (1966) *Documenta Ophthalmologica*, **20**, with permission.

circumstances one sees the expected reduction in amplitude in the presence of a dense cataract. In this same paper Burian and Burns record that coloured stimuli tend to evoke larger responses in aphakic eyes and they also observe that the duration of the 'b' wave tends to be longer pre-operatively than post-operatively (Burian and Burns, 1966). This last observation had previously been confirmed by Karpe and Vainio-Mattila (1951).

This data, together with that from several other papers written on the subject (for example see Jayle, Tassy and Graveline, 1966; Kubota and Kuroda, 1971), indicates that routine pre-operative electroretinograms on cataract patients might well be of value to the surgeon in the future. The discovery that the oscillatory potential is modified at an early stage in diabetic retinopathy will no doubt also increase the value of pre-operative electro-retinograms.

Less information is available concerning the effect of lens opacities on the visually evoked response and the electro-oculogram. Dvorak found no stat-istical difference between pre- and post-operative electro-oculograms, but there was a wide range of values in spite of repeated examinations (Dvorak, 1971).

Thompson and Harding found that cataract alone had little effect on the amplitude and latency of the flash VEP, provided that a sufficient intensity of flash was used. In their series of cataract patients they showed that the VEP proved to be an accurate predictor of visual outcome (Thompson and Hard-ing, 1978).

Opacities in the Vitreous

Vitreous opacities have been classified by Duke-Elder in the following manner (Duke-Elder, 1969):

1. Congenital remnants of the hyaloid vascular system.
2. Endogenous opacities:
   a. coagula of the colloid basis of the gel.
   b. crystalline deposits: i. asteroid bodies
                             ii. synchisis scintillans.
3. Exogenous opacities:
   a. protein coagula.
   b. exudate cells.
   c. blood.
   d. tissue cells: epithelial, histiocytic, glial.
   e. tumour cells.
   f. pigment: melanotic and haematogenous.

The most important of these types of opacity from the electrodiagnostic point of view is blood, and the discussion in this section will be limited to the management of such a case when a view of the fundus is obscured.

A vitreous haemorrhage may occur in association with the following conditions:

1. A tear of the retina.
2. Vascular disease of the retina:
   a. diabetic retinopathy.
   b. hypertensive retinopathy.
   c. central retinal vein occlusion.
   d. Eales's disease.
3. Subarachnoid haemorrhage.
4. Ocular trauma.

Retinal tears

In recent years the prophylactic treatment of retinal detachment has become more widely practised and an important aspect of this is the sealing of open breaks in the retina before they lead to a detachment. The commonest cause of these tears is contraction and detachment of the vitreous. Adhesions between the hyaloid layer of the gel and the retina are known to be particularly strong at the site of the retinal vessels and for this reason the formation of these tears is commonly followed by a vitreous haemorrhage. Usually the haemorrhage is slight, but in some cases the vision suddenly deteriorates due to more extensive bleeding. In these circumstances the surgeon may admit the patient to hospital for observation and bed rest, hoping that when the vitreous clears a flat retinal tear may become visible allowing prophylactic treatment. Sometimes after a prolonged period of bed rest a retinal detachment becomes visible. The electroretinogram changes in cases of retinal detachment are described elsewhere in this book and electroretinogram changes in eyes which have a predisposition to retinal detachment are also described. As in the case of corneal and lenticular opacities, opacities in the vitreous do not alter the electrical response from the retina to any great extent.

Vascular disease of the retina

The electroretinogram changes in diabetic retinopathy and central retinal vein occlusion are also described elsewhere in this book. In both these conditions the occurrence of a vitreous haemorrhage usually bears a poor prognosis. In cases with diabetic retinopathy recurrent haemorrhages may occur over a period of many years, the sight on each occasion being restored as the haemorrhage became absorbed (Figure 10.4). In these cases some assessment of the fundus can be made by electroretinography when the haemorrhage is dense. Eales's disease may cause vitreous haemorrhages when there is minimal vascular involvement and a normal electroretinogram can be recorded in these cases. Figure 10.5 shows the results of electroretinography in cases of vitreous haemorrhage from a variety of causes.

Now that the technique of vitrectomy is becoming more widely practised, there is a demand for more accurate testing of retinal function through opaque media. If useful results are to be obtained, it is of course essential that the stimulus should be bright enough. The superiority of the electroretinogram over other tests of retinal function in these cases has been confirmed by Fuller, Knighton and Machemer (1975).

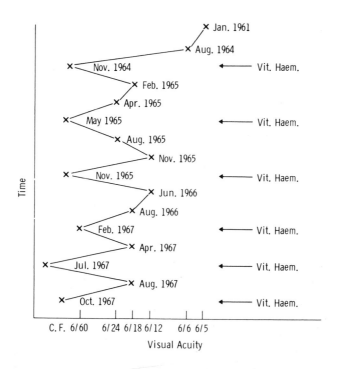

Figure 10.4. Variations in vision (without specific therapy) due to recurrent vitreous haemorrhage in a diabetic patient. Reproduced from Caird, F. I., Pirie, A. & Ramsell, T. G. (1969), in *Diabetes and the Eye*, p. 95. Oxford & Edinburgh: Blackwell Scientific Publications, with permission.

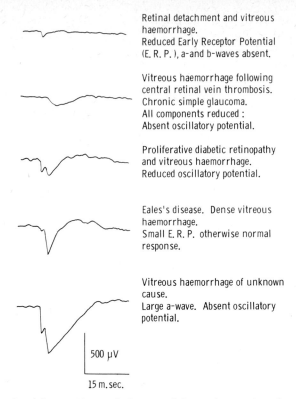

Retinal detachment and vitreous
haemorrhage.
Reduced Early Receptor Potential
(E. R. P.), a-and b-waves absent.

Vitreous haemorrhage following
central retinal vein thrombosis.
Chronic simple glaucoma.
All components reduced :
Absent oscillatory potential.

Proliferative diabetic retinopathy
and vitreous haemorrhage.
Reduced oscillatory potential.

Eales's disease. Dense vitreous
haemorrhage.
Small E. R. P. otherwise normal
response.

Vitreous haemorrhage of unknown
cause.
Large a-wave. Absent oscillatory
potential.

500 µV

15 m. sec.

Figure 10.5. Results of electroretinography in cases of vitreous haemorrhage from various causes.

Subarachnoid haemorrhage

Figure 10.6 illustrates the electroretinogram recorded simultaneously from both eyes of a 47-year-old male patient with a previous history of systemic hypertension. He was admitted unconscious to the medical ward and the diagnosis of subarachnoid haemorrhage was confirmed. On regaining consciousness he was completely blind with bilateral vitreous haemorrhages. The electroretinogram shows a normal trace in the right eye, but the oscillatory

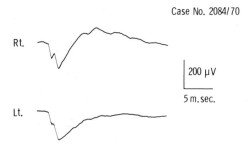

Case No. 2084/70

Rt.

200 µV

5 m. sec.

Lt.

Figure 10.6. Electroretinogram from patient with bilateral vitreous haemorrhages associated with a subarachnoid haemorrhage.

potential is absent on the left side (lower trace). The patient's name was placed on the blind register, but it was felt that the prognosis for vision was good at least for the right eye. Two years later the patient has now recovered 6/12 vision in his right eye, but the left eye remains at less than 6/60.

Ocular Trauma

Vitreous haemorrhage is a common accompaniment of perforating wounds of the globe and electroretinography may be considered after the initial healing process is complete. It would of course, be hazardous to place a contact lens electrode on to a recently perforated globe. The findings in cases of ocular trauma are also discussed elsewhere.

THE TRANSMISSION OF LIGHT THROUGH A VITREOUS HAEMORRHAGE

The finding that the presence of a cataract may actually increase the response has not so far been repeated in the case of vitreous haemorrhage, but it is perhaps just as surprising that a dense haemorrhage conducts light so well. The case of Eales's disease, whose electroretinogram is shown in Figure 10.5, had a very dense haemorrhage which obscured the red reflex. In spite of this a normal response was obtained. If we compare this with the results of placing neutral density filters in front of the stimulus light (Figure 10.7), the response is quite severely modified by a filter which causes minimal obscuration of vision. Once again we can explain this discrepancy by the light-diffusing effect of the vitreous haemorrhage.

Experiments on rabbits' eyes in which the ERG was measured after intra-vitreal injection of whole blood or haemoglobin do not seem to have shown

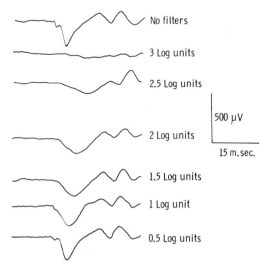

Figure 10.7. The effect of interposing different density filters in front of the stimulus flash. A normal response without a filter is shown above, and the trace using the densest filter is immediately below this.

this light-diffusing effect and only demonstrate that whole blood acts as a neutral density filter. The injection of haemoglobin appears to have some specific effect on the ERG 'b' wave (Sugita, Watanabe and Sakai, 1976).

REFERENCES

Burian, H. M. & Burns, C. A. (1966) A note on senile cataracts and the electroretinogram. *Documenta Ophthalmologica*, **20**, 141–149.

Caird, F. I., Pirie, A. & Ramsell, T. G. (1969) In *Diabetes and the Eye*, p. 95. Oxford and Edinburgh: Blackwell Scientific Publications.

Duke-Elder, Sir Stewart (1969) In *System of Ophthalmology*. Vol. XI, 5, 222. London: Henry Kimpton.

Dvorak, J. (1971) Influence of cataract extraction on the electro-oculogram. *Sbornik Lekarsky*, **73**, 166–170, No. 7 In *Ophthalmic Literature,* **25**, 4885 (1973).

Fuller, D. G., Knighton, R. W. & Machemer, R. (1975) Bright flash ERG, for evaluating eyes with opaque media. *American Journal of Ophthalmology*, **80**, 214.

Jayle, G.-E., Tassy, A. F. & Graveline, J. (1966) Electroretinogram in senile cataracts. *Vth Symposium of ISCERG (Ghent)*. In *The Clinical Value of Electroretinography*, pp. 425–434. Basel/New York: Karger. (Published 1968).

Karpe, G. & Vainio-Mattila, O. (1951) The clinical electroretinogram III: The electroretinogram in cataract. *Acta Ophthalmologica*, **29**, 113–128.

Kubota, Y. & Kuroda, N. (1971) The electroretinogram and cataract operations. *Folia Ophthalmologica Japonica*, **22**, 75–78.

Mikawa, T. & Tamura, O. (1970) Relation between the electroretinogram and post operation vision in cataract. *Japanese Journal of Clinical Ophthalmology (Rinsho Ganka)*, **24**, 43–46.

Sugita, G., Watanabe, I. & Sakai, T. (1976) ERG studies in experimental vitreous haemorrhage. *Folia Ophthalmologica Japonica*, **27**, 321–327.

Thompson, C. R. S. & Harding, G. F. A. (1978) The visual evoked response in patients with cataracts. *Documenta Ophthalmologica* (Proceedings Series), **15**, 193.

Tsinopoulos, T., Karyophyllis, K. & Konstas, P. (1972) Electroretinography in the detection of the functional condition of the retina in cataract. *Archives of the Ophthalmological Society of Northern Greece*, **18**, 69–74. In *Ophthalmic Literature*, **26**, 779 (1972).

CHAPTER ELEVEN

Electrodiagnostic Tests in Toxic and Deficiency States

A considerable amount of information is now available about the effect of various drugs on the electrical responses from the eye. This data has been provided both by animal experiments and by the results of overdosage or accidental ingestion in human subjects. Electrodiagnostic tests have been applied in such circumstances to find out more about the nature and origin of the response and in some cases to help make a diagnosis. These techniques are also being used in an attempt to localise the site of action of drugs in the eye. Undoubtedly the nature of these electrical changes is such that they can carry useful objective clinical information, but our knowledge is still very limited and the results must be interpreted with great care. In spite of the fact that the International Society for Clinical Electrophysiology of Vision (ISCEV) aims to integrate clinical and laboratory studies, there is surprisingly little overlap between the drugs tested on animals and those used on humans. In this chapter it is intended to consider first some of the results of animal experiments and then to discuss toxicity in the human.

ANIMAL STUDIES

For many years much interest has been centred on the use of drugs to produce selective damage to different layers of the retina. It was hoped that corresponding changes in the electroretinogram would provide information about the origin of its different components. Considerable encouragement to this approach was given by Noell when he showed that sodium iodate, which selectively damages the pigment epithelium, abolishes the 'c' wave in rabbits (Noell, 1953). This was such a clear-cut example of selective action of a drug with corresponding changes in the electroretinogram that it has become accepted as a classical study, but the problem is probably rather more complex. For example, there is quite good evidence that in the human the 'c' wave is abolished at least in part by the use of miotics or mydriatics, suggesting that the 'c' wave may have a pupillociliary origin (Pearlman, 1962). It also seems likely that the action of sodium iodate is not as selective as was once believed. For these reasons this type of localisation work is being superseded by micro-electrode experiments. In a recent study the toxic effects of sodium iodate were examined with the electron microscope and it seems that although selective damage to the pigment epithelium and the outer segments of the receptors is first seen, this damage extends inwards over a period of hours to involve the whole retina. If the electroretinogram is monitored during this period it is interesting that there is an initial increase in the size of both 'a' and 'b' waves, but these become extinguished as the inner parts of the retina become degenerate. The electro-oculogram on the other hand becomes affected within an hour, the light rise is reduced and the transient becomes reversed. The electrodiagnostic changes reflect the inward spread of retinal damage (Imaizumi, Tazawa and Kobayashi, 1972).

Another substance which has been used for localisation studies is sodium L-glutamate. This causes loss of vision in mice and selective loss of the inner layers of the retina with destruction of the bipolars and ganglion cells (Lucas and Newhouse, 1957). When it is injected into rabbits or rats, the 'b' wave becomes depressed after three months and eventually can be seen as a small hump at the peak of the 'a' wave. This is probably a delayed effect because after a single large dose of glutamate both 'a' and 'b' waves become reduced for the first days and then increase again. The electro-oculogram is also affected at this early stage. In theory at least one would not expect the electro-oculogram or the 'a' wave to be affected by a drug which only damaged the inner layers of the retina, but the experimental results do not all agree on this and perhaps the lesion produced by sodium glutamate can vary with dosage (Hamatsu, 1964; Buckser and Buckser, 1971; Imaizumi, Tazawa and Kobayashi, 1972).

The injection of azide into experimental animals produces changes in the standing potential as well as the 'c' wave which have led people to believe that it has a specific effect on the pigment epithelium. In this instance as well, however, more recent work has revealed changes in the 'a' and 'b' waves as well as the oscillatory potential (Takeda, 1965; Francois, Jonsas and De Rouck, 1969a).

A wide variety of other substances has been tested; for example it has been shown that insulin produces generalised changes in the electroretinogram which may indicate the widespread effect of hypoglycaemia on the retina (Francois, Jonsas and De Rouck, 1969b; Honda, 1971). An important field is the study of the effects of anaesthesia on the electrical response. Pentobarbitone reduces the size of the oscillatory potential in rabbits but at lower dosage levels the electrical response may be increased (Takeda, 1966; Trimarchi, 1968). In clinical practice routine electroretinography and electro-oculography are performed under general anaesthesia, and we assume that anaesthesia has no effect on the response for these purposes. Our knowledge of the effect of anaesthesia on the human electroretinogram is very limited; obviously it is not feasible to collect a 'normal' series but undoubtedly completely normal responses are often seen. The oscillatory potential for example does not appear to be affected by the dose of anaesthetic used in the operating theatre.

One might expect the pattern VEP to be abolished by general anaesthesia, although this subject does not appear to have been studied. The flash VEP can be recorded under general anaesthesia but the exact effect of the anaesthetic on the amplitude is also not known (Wright, Arden and Jones, 1973).

A comprehensive list of all the drugs which have been tested for their effects on the electrical response from the retina would be of doubtful value but Table 11.1 gives a sample of some of these together with their effects.

Table 11.1. Effect of some drugs on the electroretinogram

Drug	Effect on electroretinogram	Author
Ethyl alcohol	'b' wave increase	Manfredini and Trimarchi (1968) Levett and Morini (1978)
Amyl acetate	Progressive reduction of 'a' and 'b' waves but return to normal after 45 days	Gorgone et al (1970)
Dichlorophenamide	55 per cent increase in 'b' wave	Tota and Cavallacci (1970)
Carbon disulphide	Rapid and irreversible extinction of 'a' and 'b' waves	Malfitono et al (1972)
Triamterene	'b' wave increased by 40 per cent in rabbits	Tota and Cavallacci (1971)
Strychnine	'b' wave increased but lowered in higher concentrations in rabbit	Vörkel and Hanitzsch (1971)
Alpha-chymotrypsin	Reduction of 'b' wave; appearance of slow wavelets	Yoshito et al (1972)

CLINICAL STUDIES

The Antimalarials

Quinine

Although the toxic effects of quinine have been well recognised for many years, there still exists a controversy as to the exact mode of action of this poison and electrodiagnostic tests help to throw some light on the problem. An overdose of quinine is usually taken in an attempt to procure an abortion but cases have been reported in which an overdose was ingested as a prophylactic for malaria (Stein, 1970). Symptoms may follow after taking as little as one gram in sensitive individuals, but the usual dose to cause blindness is put at 2.5 to 4 g. The affected patient experiences deafness, tinnitus, and visual failure and larger doses produce coma. The fundus appearance may be normal at first, but in some cases there is retinal oedema with a cherry red spot at the macula. The visual fields become grossly constricted. The symptoms and signs often improve over a period of weeks and the fundus then begins to show optic atrophy and narrowing of the retinal arteries (Berggren and Rendahl, 1955; Bard and Gills, 1964).

For many years arguments have been put forward to decide whether the toxic effect of quinine is primarily on the retinal vessels or whether it has a

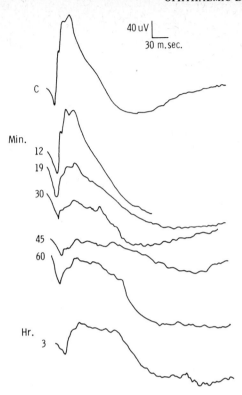

Figure 11.1. Electroretinographic tracings taken prior to (C) and after oral administration of quinine. An increase in the size of the 'a' wave is accompanied by reduction of the 'b' wave. The changes show recovery after 45 minutes. Reproduced from Cibis, Burian & Blodi (1973) Electroretinogram changes in acute quinine poisoning. *Archives of Ophthalmology*, **40**, 307. Copyright 1973 American Medical Association, with permission of authors and editor.

direct toxic effect on the retina. The question of vascular spasm is not easy to answer because we know that almost any condition which causes optic atrophy also causes constriction of the retinal vessels. Investigation of the effect of acute poisoning in animals has shown that the electroretinogram is initially depressed but recovers in a matter of hours (Figure 11.1). After this a further slow deterioration in the response occurs, but the relatively slight degree of these changes compared with the severe visual loss indicates primary damage to the ganglion cell and nerve fibre layer (Hommer, 1968). In humans the electroretinogram may show a gradual decline between ten days and ten months after intoxication, and paradoxically the vision may be gradually improving during this period (Figure 11.2). The electro-oculogram has shown an absent light rise during the first few days after intoxication and this has then recovered in parallel with the subjective improvement (Figure 11.3) (Behrman and Mushin, 1968). The absence of a light rise on the electro-oculogram is not easy to explain in terms of a ganglion cell poison and more cases will have to be investigated in detail in future in order to find the true answer to this conflicting evidence. The matter takes on more clinical import-

VISUAL FIELDS   ELECTRORETINOGRAM

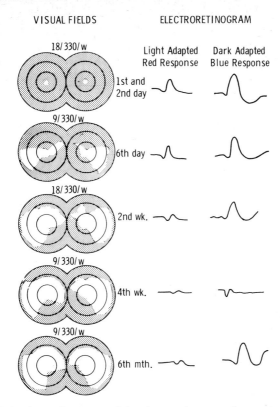

Figure 11.2. Diminution and recovery of the electroretinogram after acute quinine poisoning. Reproduced from Bard & Gills (1964) Quinine amblyopia. *Archives of Ophthalmology*, **72**, 328. Copyright 1964 American Medical Association, with permission of authors and editor.

ance when we consider that disseminated sclerosis can present in a young girl in a rather similar manner; the fundus in bilateral optic neuritis may be completely normal and then gradually vision recovers in association with optic atrophy and narrowing of the retinal vessels.

Chloroquine (resochin)

Chloroquine was used extensively but in small doses in the war years as a prophylactic treatment for malaria. Corneal changes resulting from this drug were described at the end of the war, but the more serious retinotoxic effects were not observed until large doses were employed in the treatment of disseminated lupus erythematosus and rheumatoid arthritis. Its value in the treatment of disseminated lupus erythematosus was described in 1954 and the first case of chloroquine retinopathy was described in 1957 (Cambiaggi, 1957). Since then reports from many different centres have confirmed that when the total dose of chloroquine exceeds 100 g there is a high risk of visual disturbance with associated changes in the fundus. The earliest sign of retinopathy is a perimacular pigmentary desturbance described as a 'bull's eye appearance' (Henkind, Carr and Siegel, 1964). In more advanced cases the arteries became

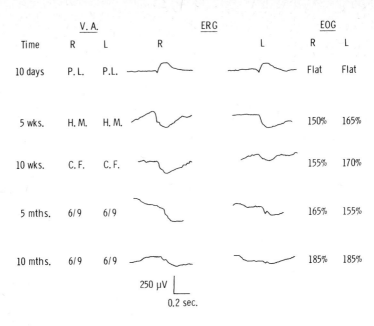

Figure 11.3. Changes in visual acuity, electroretinogram and electro-oculogram after quinine intoxication in man. Reproduced from Behrman & Mushin (1968) Electrodiagnostic findings in quinine amblyopia. *British Journal of Ophthalmology*, **52**, 925, with permission of authors and editor.

attenuated and peripheral pigmentation may appear. By the time that fundus changes appear, irreversible field defects can be detected and in some cases a progressive deterioration of vision occurs in spite of cessation of treatment. Histopathological investigation of human eyes and animal experiments have shown that chloroquine accumulates in and damages the receptor layer and the pigment epithelium, thus confirming the cumulative nature of the toxicity (Wetterholm and Winter, 1964).

Electroretinographic studies have shown a depression of the 'b' wave amplitude in patients who have had treatment for more than a year, but in some series the electroretinogram was normal in the presence of fundus changes (Schmidt and Muller Limmroth, 1962; Henkind, Carr and Siegel, 1964). It does appear that the electroretinogram may be of some prognostic value in these cases. This has been shown in a long-term follow-up study of fifteen cases of chloroquine poisoning (Kubota, Kubota and Asanigi, 1978). The changes in the electro-oculogram were first described by Arden in 1962 (Arden and Fojas, 1962). In a detailed study Kolb showed that depression of the light rise of the electro-oculogram is often an early sign of toxicity which may sometimes precede the fundus changes. In a series of 47 cases there was considerable overlap between treated and non-treated results (Figure 11.4). Furthermore, it was shown that in a group of patients who had not received treatment but who suffered from collagen disease, the mean value of the Arden Index was below normal, but not so low as in the group that had been treated with chloroquine. A study of patients in whom the drug therapy had

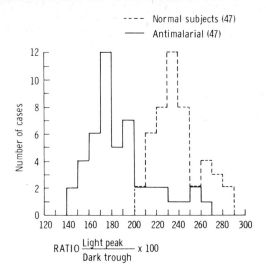

Figure 11.4. The Arden Index for 47 normal subjects and 47 patients treated with chloroquine. Reproduced from Kolb, H. (1965) Electro-oculogram findings in patients treated with anti-malarial drugs. *British Journal of Ophthalmology*, **49**, 573, with permission of author and editor.

been stopped revealed a return to normal of the Arden Index in many cases (Kolb, 1965).

Both chloroquine and hydroxychloroquine (Plaquenil) produce the same toxic effects but the toxic and the normal dose of hydroxychloroquine is much larger. The evidence now indicates clearly that these drugs should not be used if at all possible and if they are used the patients should be carefully monitored by an ophthalmologist. If the electro-oculogram is depressed then the drug should be stopped even if there are no subjective signs of toxicity. Unfortunately there is no doubt that some patients may develop severe toxicity with a normal electro-oculogram. Figure 11.5 shows the results obtained from a patient on chloroquine. The patient had complained of the appearance of a dark 'blob' in front of her vision and was advised to stop using the drug on the strength of the electrodiagnostic findings.

In spite of its obvious hazards, chloroquine is still being prescribed in this country. Recently it has been found useful in short courses for the treatment of pulmonary sarcoidosis and ophthalmologists must be continually on their guard for the appearance of side effects.

Case 1.

Electrooculogram

Figure 11.5. Case 1. Reduced light rise in patient treated with Plaquenil for 18 months. Arden Index—R 157 per cent. L 144 per cent. Vision R 6/12: L 6/9. Fundi doubtful changes at right macula. Aged 62 years.

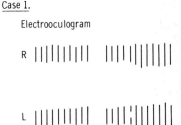

Phenothiazines

Many derivatives of phenothiazine are now used in medical practice as tranquillisers and they can be divided into three groups:

1. *Dimethylamines*. This group includes chlorpromazine (Largactil) and promazine (Sparine). It is doubtful if either of these drugs are retinotoxic, although chlorpromazine is known to produce characteristic lens opacities as well as opacities in the cornea. In a series of 462 patients receiving chlorpromazine no cases of retinal involvement could be found, and although only a few electro-oculograms were performed the results were all within normal limits (Mathalone, 1967).

2. *Piperidines*. This group includes the drug NP 207, which was never marketed because of its retinotoxicity. An extensive clinical trial was sufficient to produce fundus changes resembling retinitis pigmentosa as well as corresponding changes in the electroretinogram (Goar and Fletcher, 1956). Thioridazin (Melleril) is also included in this group and this has also been shown to be retinotoxic but only in high doses.

3. *Piperazines*. Under this heading are included prochlorperazine (Stemetil), and trifluoperazine (Stelazine). No retinal disturbances have been described after the use of drugs in this third group.

Although the evidence is limited, it would appear that electrodiagnostic studies do not provide an early indication of phenothiazine retinopathy at least in their present form. In an investigation in The Netherlands of 93 patients on these drugs, only 34 per cent of those showing a retinopathy had abnormal electro-oculograms (Boet, 1970; Cohen, Wells and Borda, 1978).

Vitamin A Deficiency

It has been seen in a previous chapter that many conditions which cause night blindness tend to cause marked alterations in the electrical response of the eye to light. It is perhaps not surprising that vitamin A deficiency also causes severe impairment of the scotopic electroretinogram and may abolish the light rise of the electro-oculogram. These changes may be reversed by treatment (Tamaki, 1968; Gombos, Hornblass and Vendeland, 1970). A case of particular significance was recently reported. It concerned a 25-year-old male patient who had deliberately eaten a vitamin A-free diet as supposed treatment for grand mal epilepsy. He refused any treatment of his eyes until severe symptoms and signs had appeared. Before treatment the scotopic electroretinogram was markedly reduced and there was no detectable light rise on electro-oculography. Dark adaptation was also grossly abnormal and scattered yellow dots were visible in the fundus. Blood levels of vitamin A were abnormally low. Seven weeks after treatment had been started, the electroretinogram showed only a slight abnormality in the scotopic response and the Arden Index was 133 per cent R and 114 per cent L. After three months the fundi were normal and after eleven months the Arden Index read 130 per cent R and 150 per cent L. Dark adaptation remained grossly abnormal after eleven months (Bors and Fells, 1971).

Other Drugs which Produce Electrical Changes

The possibility that the eye and in particular the retina might be a sensitive sentinel of drug toxicity has led to the investigation of many different drugs. Lead poisoning, for example, may produce severe electroretinographic changes at an early stage (Guguchkova, 1972). Indomethacin has also been incriminated as a cause of chloroquine-like changes both in the cornea and the retina and alterations of the electroretinogram have been described (Burns, 1968). The introduction of ethambutol in the treatment of tuberculosis has been associated with oedema of the macula and optic neuritis. In a series of six patients treated for one year no electrodiagnostic abnormalities were observed. Figure 11.6 shows the results from a patient who had been treated for two years with ethambutol for pulmonary tuberculosis. He began complaining of blurring of his vision and was found to have macula oedema. The electroretinogram is normal for his age, but the electro-oculogram is considerably reduced.

Electroretinography and electro-oculography undoubtedly have a part to play in the investigation of toxic and deficiency states both in the laboratory and in the clinic, but as with so many other applications of these techniques their value is limited by a lack of knowledge of the significance of the results. The place of the visual evoked response in the investigation of, for example, psychotropic drugs, or drugs causing optic nerve damage, has yet to be ascertained.

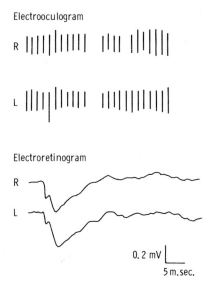

Figure 11.6. Recording from a patient treated with ethambutol for two years. Electro-oculogram: Arden Index—R 165 per cent. L 140 per cent. (Normal—above 170 per cent). Electroretinogram: 'a' and 'b' waves within normal limits for age of patient. Small wavelets but within normal limits for age.

REFERENCES

Arden, G. B. & Fojas, M. R. (1962) Electrophysiological abnormalities in pigmentary degenerations of the retina. *Archives of Ophthalmology*, **68**, 369.

Bard, L. A. & Gills, J. P. (1964) Quinine amblyopia. *Archives of Ophthalmology*, **72**, 328.

Behrman, J. & Mushin, A. (1968) Electrodiagnostic findings in quinine amblyopia. *British Journal of Ophthalmology*, **52**, 925.

Berggren, L. & Rendahl, I. (1955) Electroretinogram in quinine poisoning. *Acta Ophthalmologica*, **33**, 217.

Boet, D. J. (1970) Toxic effects of phenothiazines. *Documenta Ophthalmologica*, **28**, 1–69.

Bors, F. & Fells, P. (1971) Reversal of the complications of self-induced vitamin A deficiency. *British Journal of Ophthalmology*, **55**, 210.

Buckser, S. & Buckser, C. (1971) Effect of sodium glutamate on the electroretinogram. *American Journal of Ophthalmology*, **48**, 504–521.

Burns, C. A. (1968) Indomethacin, reduced retinal sensitivity and corneal deposits. *American Journal of Ophthalmology*, **66**, 825–835.

Cambiaggi, A. (1957) Unusual ocular lesions in a case of systemic lupus erythematosis. *Archives of Ophthalmology*, **57**, 451.

Cibis, G., Burian, H. & Blodi, F. C. (1973) Electroretinogram changes in acute quinine poisoning. *Archives of Ophthalmology*, **40**, 307.

Cohen, J., Wells, J. & Borda, R. (1978) Thioridazine (Mellaril) ocular toxicity. *Documenta Ophthalmologica* (Proceedings Series), **15**, 91.

Francois, J., Jonsas, C. & De Rouck, A. (1969a) Experimental studies of the effect of sodium azide on the electroretinogram and the electro-oculogram in rabbits. *Anales del Instituto Barraquer*, **9**, 293–298.

Francois, J., Jonsas, C. & De Rouck, A. (1969b) Experimental studies of the effect of hypoglycaemia. *Annals of Ophthalmology*, **1**, 66–71.

Goar, E. L. & Fletcher, M. C. (1956) Toxic chorioretinopathy following the use of NP 207. *Transactions of the American Ophthalmological Society*, **54**, 129–139.

Gombos, G., Hornblass, A. & Vendeland, J. (1970) Ocular manifestations of vitamin A deficiency. *Annals of Ophthalmology*, **2**, 680–684.

Gorgone, G., Inserra, A., Barlotta, F. & Malfitano, D. (1970) Electroretinogram in experimental intoxication with amyl acetate. *Annali di Ottalmologie e Clinica Oculista*, **96**, 313–319.

Guguchkova, P. T. (1972) Electroretinogram and electro-oculogram examination of people occupationally exposed to the effects of lead over a long period. *Vestnik Oftalmologii*, **85**, 60–65.

Hamatsu, T. (1964) Effect of sodium iodate and sodium L-glutamate on the rabbit retina. *Acta Societatis Ophthalmologicae Japonicae*, **68**, 1621–1636.

Henkind, P., Carr, R. E. & Siegel, I. M. (1964) Early chloroquine retinopathy: clinical and functional findings. *Archives of Ophthalmology*, **71**, 157.

Hommer, K. (1968) Über die Chininvergiftung der Netzhaut mit einer Bermerkung zür experimentellen Chlorochinvergiftung. *Klinische Monatsblätter für Augenheilkunde*, **152**, 785–805.

Honda, Y. (1971) The mode of action of insulin upon the electrical activity of mammalian retinas in vitro. *Experientia*, **27**, 395.

Imaizumi, K., Tazawa, Y. & Kobayashi, H. (1972) Electrophysiological and histopathological studies on the rabbit retina treated with sodium iodate and sodium L-glutamate. *Xth ISCERG Symposium, Los Angeles*. The Hague: Dr. W. Junk, B.V.

Kolb, H. (1965) Electro-oculogram findings in patients treated with antimalarial drugs. *British Journal of Ophthalmology*, **49**, 573.

Kubota, Y., Kubota, S. & Asanigi, (1978) The ERG of chloroquine in clinical retinopathy: The prognostic significance of abnormalities on the ERG. *Documenta Ophthalmologica* (Proceedings Series), **15**, 95.

Levett, J. & Morini, F. (1978) The influence of ethanol on retinal oscillatory potentials. *Documenta Ophthalmologica* (Proceedings Series), **15**, 133.

Lucas, D. R. & Newhouse, J. P. (1957) The toxic effect of sodium L-glutamate on the inner layers of the retina. *Archives of Ophthalmology*, **58**, 193–201.

Malfitano, D., Barlotta, F., Inserra, A. & Gorgone, G. (1972) Electroretinographic findings following experimental poisoning with carbon disulphide. *Bolletino della Società di Biologia Sperimentale*, **48**, 113–115.

Manfredini, U. & Trimarchi, F. (1968) L'azione dell'alcool etilico sull' electroretinogramma. *Annali di Ottalmologia e Clinica Oculista*, **94**, 155–160.

Mathalone, M. B. R. (1967) Eye and skin changes in psychiatric patients treated with chlorpromazine. *British Journal of Ophthalmology*, **51**, 86.

Noell, W. K. (1953) Experimentally induced toxic effects on structure and function of visual cells and pigment epithelium. *American Journal of Ophthalmology*, **36**, 103–116.

Pearlman, J. (1962) The 'c' wave of the human electroretinogram. *Archives of Ophthalmology*, **68**, 823–830.

Schmidt, B. & Muller Limmroth, W. (1962) Electroretinographic examinations following the application of chloroquine. *Acta Ophthalmologica*, Supp. **70**, 245–251.

Stein, H. J. (1970) Das Elektroretinogramm bei der Chinin-Intoxikation: Ein Beitrag zür Genese der Retinitis pigmentosa. *Medizinische Welt*, **21**, 774–778.

Takeda, H. (1965) Effects of azide on the electroretinogram and standing potential in the rabbit eye. *Acta Societas Ophthalmologicae Japonicae*, **69**, 1187–1195.

Takeda, H. (1966) Effect of Nembutal on the electroretinogram of the rabbit eye. *Acta Societas Ophthalmologicae Japonicae*, **70**, 2171–2175.

Tamaki, S. (1968) Electroretinographic studies of experimental hypervitaminosis A and vitamin A deficiency, report IV; The influence of vitamin A deficiency and light adaptation on the electroretinogram of rats. *Acta Societas Ophthalmologicae Japonicae*, **72**, 1209.

Tota, G. & Cavallacci, G. (1970) Changes in the electroretinogram produced by dichlorophenamide. *Annali di Ottalmologie e Clinica Oculista*, **96**, 303–311.

Tota, G. & Cavallacci, G. (1971) The electroretinogram after administration of triamterene. *Annali di Ottalmologie e Clinica Oculista*, **97**, 143–153.

Trimarchi, F. (1968) L'azione dei barbiturici sull'elettroretinogramma. *Annali di Ottalmologie e Clinica Oculista*, **94**, 1225–1229.

Vörkel, W. & Hanitzsch, R. (1971) Effect of strychnine on the electroretinogram of the isolated rabbit retina. *Experimentia*, **27**, 296–297.

Wetterholm, D. H. & Winter, F. C. (1964) Histopathology of chloroquine retinal toxicity. *Archives of Ophthalmology*, **71**, 82.

Wright, J., Arden, G. & Jones, B. R. (1973) Continuous monitoring of the VER during surgery. *Transactions of the Ophthalmological Society of the United Kingdom*, **93**, 311.

CHAPTER TWELVE

The Effect of Injury

Electrodiagnostic tests have two clear advantages over the other accepted techniques that are readily available for examining the eye. Firstly, they can give information about the retina when the media have become opaque, and secondly, they give a result which can be measured objectively. The information that these tests can provide depends entirely on the available data and it is unfortunate that our knowledge of the behaviour of the response in disease and injury is often rather scanty. This applies particularly in the field of trauma where the amount of clinical information collected to date is very limited.

This might seem surprising when one considers that the need for information about the retina is particularly important in these cases. The younger age groups are often involved and medico-legal implications may demand a very accurate prognosis. But there are technical difficulties which may discourage the clinician from employing electrodiagnostic tests. It is not feasible to fit a contact lens electrode to an eye which has recently suffered a perforating wound, for obvious reasons. In the early stages after an injury the patient is often confined to bed, whether because of his eye or because of injuries elsewhere, and it may not be considered practical to transfer him to the electrodiagnostic clinic.

Many of these difficulties can be overcome by using special techniques. For example, cotton wick electrodes may be used, or hook-shaped eyelid retractors made of silver have been found to be effective. These electrodes tend to produce a smaller response than standard contact lens electrodes and the background noise is sometimes more marked. However, by averaging a small number of the responses, a clear-cut result should be obtained. The difficulty of moving the patient can be overcome by the use of portable equipment. Electronic equipment of all types has become smaller and lighter over the years and although ophthalmic electrodiagnostic equipment is still rather bulky it is to be hoped that improvements will continue to occur in the future.

In spite of these drawbacks it will be seen in this chapter that electrodiagnostic tests can give us useful information about the extent of an injury and the onset of complicating features such as retinal detachment, sympathetic ophthalmitis or ocular metallosis.

CONTUSION INJURIES AND PERFORATING WOUNDS

As a general rule the electro-oculogram is more severely affected by injury than the electroretinogram. For example, after blunt trauma the electro-oculogram is depressed for a few days if the injury is slight and permanently in severe cases. The 'a' wave of the electroretinogram is only depressed after severe injuries whereas the 'b' wave may show some depression after light blunt injuries (Gliem, Moller and Keitzman, 1971). Permanent changes in the electro-oculogram and electroretinogram reflect permanent changes in the retina.

The prognostic value of these tests can only be assessed by the investigation of large series of patients with adequate follow-up. A series of 32 eyes were followed long enough for their final visual acuity to be determined. The results were divided into four groups according to the size of the electroretinogram recorded within two months after the injury. They were classified simply as 'extinguished', 'greatly diminished', 'subnormal' and 'normal'. The final recovery was assessed when the eye had settled completely and when any cataract present had been removed. All the eyes in the 'extinguished' group were for practical purposes blind, and three had to be eviscerated or enucleated. Nine out of ten eyes with a normal electroretinogram made a good recovery and the remaining one developed a retinal detachment. The electroretinogram helped to diagnose this. In the intermediate groups the responses were scattered in a manner consistent with the group (Jayle, Tassy and Ghnassia, 1970). A larger series of 64 eyes in 60 patients has since served to confirm the prognostic value of electrodiagnostic tests; in this series both the ERG and VEP results were combined to give the best prognostic value. A skin ERG showing reduction of 'b' wave amplitude of less than 50 per cent and a VEP with amplitude reduction, also less than 50 per cent without latency delay, invariably predicted a good visual prognosis. In five cases in this series with enucleated eyes and retina *in situ* the electrophysiological findings correlated well with the histology (Crews, Thompson and Harding 1978).

The results of other investigations along these lines seem to confirm that the modification of the electroretinogram is proportional to the extent of damage to the retina. When the response is extinguished the prognosis is nearly always poor. This is important when the risk of sympathetic ophthalmitis raises the question of enucleation. An extinguished electroretinogram at this point will allow the surgeon to proceed with enucleation in the knowledge that the eye is unlikely to recover any vision.

Figure 12.1 shows the electro-oculogram from a patient who was admitted with a hyphaema after a lump of soil had been thrown into his eye. Because he developed secondary glaucoma, the anterior chamber was washed out, but at the time of discharge he had a dense vitreous haemorrhage and the prognosis was uncertain. It can be seen that the Arden Index is within normal limits in both eyes. The fact that the size of the bars for the right eye are smaller than those on the left is not significant. Figure 12.2 shows the electro-

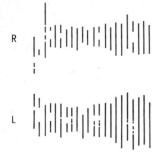

R

L

Figure 12.1. Electro-oculogram taken five months after contusion injury to right eye. Fundus view obscured by vitreous haemorrhage. Arden Index: 220 per cent R. & L.

retinogram obtained from a patient who was an inmate of one of the local prisons. He had been struck in the eye by someone's boot and had claimed that the eye was completely blind since then. There was no evidence of injury and the electroretinogram was normal. More important information in this case was provided by the visually evoked response. This was also quite normal for each eye. The visually evoked response has a particular part to play in contusion injuries in view of the occasional occurrence of severe damage to the optic nerve after a relatively trivial injury. The clinician is sometimes surprised to find that an eye is completely blind when initial traumatic swelling of the lids has subsided. The pupil is nearly always dilated and fails to react to direct light but at this stage the optic disc is not atrophic. The prognosis for vision is usually very poor in the affected eye, but occasionally one can be surprised by the amount of recovery that occurs. Perhaps the visually evoked response will in the future be able to help us assess the amount of permanent damage in these cases.

Figure 12.3 shows the result of electro-oculography performed two weeks and three months after a contusion injury to the right eye. The patient had a total hyphaema, a vitreous haemorrhage and secondary glaucoma. Light projection was difficult to assess. At first the Arden Index was severely reduced and a retinal detachment was suspected but this showed a dramatic recovery in spite of a persistent vitreous haemorrhage. The patient's vision has since gradually recovered and the initial poor response must have been due to the direct effect of contusion of the retina.

Figure 12.2. Electroretinogram from both eyes three weeks after claimed contusion injury to left eye. Visual acuity: R—6/6, L—P of L.

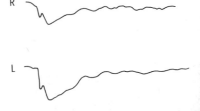

R

L

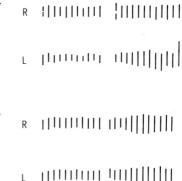

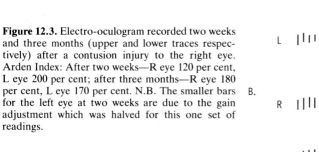

Figure 12.3. Electro-oculogram recorded two weeks and three months (upper and lower traces respectively) after a contusion injury to the right eye. Arden Index: After two weeks—R eye 120 per cent, L eye 200 per cent; after three months—R eye 180 per cent, L eye 170 per cent. N.B. The smaller bars for the left eye at two weeks are due to the gain adjustment which was halved for this one set of readings.

OCULAR METALLOSIS

Although our knowledge of the electrical response of the eye following perforating and contusion injuries is limited, there has been a considerable interest both in the clinic and in the laboratory in the problem of diagnosing ocular metallosis.

Metal particles lodged in the vitreous have a specific toxic effect on the tissues which depends on the particular metal concerned. The nature of the metal, its alloy content and the degree of encapsulation in the tissues are all factors which may determine the type of reaction shown by the eye. Copper is less corrosive than iron but it is more toxic to the retina; aluminium is less corrosive than either of these and is also less toxic. Ocular metallosis is characterised clinically by brown pigmentation of the iris, lens capsule and vitreous with contraction of the visual fields and progressive night blindness.

It was Karpe who originally demonstrated the changes in the electroretinogram in siderosis and since then several different workers have confirmed and expanded the original findings (Karpe, 1948). It is now widely accepted that the first change to be seen is an increase in the size of the 'a' wave producing a 'negative plus' type of response. Subsequently the size of the 'b' wave diminishes giving a 'negative minus' type of response and finally the electroretinogram becomes extinguished (Figure 12.4). In another study of 68 cases the negative minus group was further subdivided into three stages and it was suggested that stage II marked a critical point beyond which the prognosis became very poor (Knave, 1969).

It would appear that the negative plus type of response is a very early change and in some series it was not observed, In animal experiments it was not seen after intravitreal implantation of copper wire into rats' eyes, but the increase in amplitude of the 'a' wave could have been masked in these instances by urethane anaesthesia (Schmidt and Weber, 1970).

If doubt has been cast on the significance of this initial negative plus response, there seems little doubt that the scotopic activity of the electro-

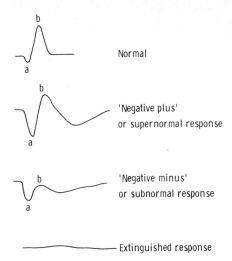

Figure 12.4. Diagram to show the three types of response which have been described at different stages in the development of siderosis oculi.

retinogram is impaired first and that the photopic activity is more resistant. Furthermore, it has been shown that the electro-oculogram is a sensitive indicator of ocular metallosis, being affected before both photopic and scotopic responses of the electroretinogram (Francois et al, 1972).

Figure 12.5 shows the electroretinogram and electro-oculogram from a patient who had a metallic foreign body encapsulated within the lens of his left eye. The lens was cataractous and the surgeon wished to know whether there was evidence of metallosis in the retina before removing the cataract. All the responses are within normal limits. The slightly reduced electro-oculogram on the left side was not significant and cataract surgery was successful.

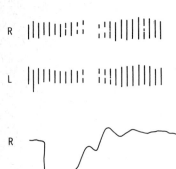

Figure 12.5. Electroretinogram and electro-oculogram from a patient who had a metallic foreign body encapsulated in the lens of his left eye. Arden Index: R—200 per cent, L—190 per cent. Electroretinogram normal response.

The medico-legal value of the VEP has been stressed in post-traumatic cases. Visual disturbances following head injury are common and sometimes they are found in the absence of clinical signs of residual injury. Absent VEPs have been demonstrated in some of these patients (Feinsod et al, 1976). One might hope that the VEP could give some indication of the prognosis in patients following injury or cerebral vascular disease, and some attempts have been made to show this.

REFERENCES

Crews, S. J., Thompson, C. R. S. & Harding, G. P. A. (1978) The ERG and VEP in patients with severe eye injury. *Documenta Ophthalmologica* (Proceedings Series), **15**.

Feinsod, M., Hoyt, W., Wilson, B. & Spire, J. P. (1976) Visually evoked response: Use in neurologic evaluation of post-traumatic subjective visual complaints. *Archives of Ophthalmology* (Chicago), **94**, 237.

Francois, J., De Rouck, A., Tacite, D. A. & Scarpulla, B. (1972) Ocular metallosis. *VIIth ISCERG Symposium*, pp. 251–267. Pisa: Pacini.

Gliem, H., Möller, D. E. & Kietzmann, G. (1971) The prognostic value of ERG and EOG in blunt contusion of the globe. *Ophthalmologica (Basel)*, **163**, No. 6, 411–417.

Jayle, G. E., Tassy, A. F. & Ghnassia, J. P. (1967) Intérêt pronostique de l'éléctrorétinogramme dans les traumatismes oculaires graves récents avec fond d'oeil invisible. *Bulletin des Sociétés d'Ophthalmologie de France (Paris)*, **67**, 685–690.

Karpe, G. (1948) Early diagnosis of siderosis retinae for the use of electroretinography. *Documenta Ophthalmalogica (Den Haag)*, **2**, 277–296.

Knave, B. (1969) Electroretinography in eye with retained intraocular metallic foreign bodies. A clinical study. *Acta Ophthalmologica (Kobenhavn)*, Suppl. **100**, 1–66.

Schmidt, J. G. H. & Weber, E. (1972) The effect of intra-ocular copper alloys on the electroretinogram of human and rat retinas. *VIIth ISCERG Symposium, 1970*, pp. 240–250. Pisa: Pacini.

CHAPTER THIRTEEN

The Scope of Electrodiagnosis in Ophthalmology

The function of the electrodiagnostic clinic in an eye hospital could be summarised as follows: it involves the measurement of two important bioelectric potentials, the corneo-retinal potential and the scalp potentials over the occipital lobes of the brain. The first of these is measured by electroretinography and electro-oculography and the second by the visually evoked potential.

In the light of the foregoing chapters, let us consider how these measurements can be of most use to the clinical ophthalmologist. It is important to realise that in most instances one measurement is not sufficient without the other. The electroretinogram and electro-oculogram both give us information about the state of the retina but tell us nothing about the ganglion cells or the remainder of the visual pathway. The visually evoked potential can give us information about the ganglion cells and the rest of the visual pathway but can only be accurately interpreted if we know about the function of the rest of the retina. The visually evoked potential measures the end result of visual processing so that it may be disturbed by a lesion anywhere in the visual pathway including the retina. At the same time it is extremely sensitive to relatively subtle changes in visual function. The electroretinogram and the electro-oculogram provide a more crude measure of visual function if one is thinking of their relationship to the act of seeing and visual acuity but they can be a sensitive index of early diffuse retinal disease, retinal toxicity or ischaemia.

The following types of cases can most usefully be referred to the electrodiagnostic clinic: any patients with densely opaque media; patients with abnormally pigmented fundi; patients with optic atrophy of unknown cause; patients with suspected hysterical amblyopia; and cases where one wishes to monitor the toxicity of certain drugs. In fact an electrodiagnostic examination is advisable in almost any instance where the diagnosis is in doubt.

The reader of this book will now realise that although much of the data obtained by these tests is of considerable clinical value there are still very many questions to be answered and it is important that the electrodiagnostic clinic pursues some line of research. Some of the avenues to be explored can be placed under the following headings:

1. *Investigations into the origin of the waveform*

Much of the recent work on the waveform of the electroretinogram has entailed the use of microelectrodes and has therefore been confined to animal experiments. Careful studies of the effect of specific diseases in humans on the waveform of the electroretinogram are still needed. The field for investigating the waveform of the visually evoked potential seems to be wide open to anyone interested.

2. *Investigation of the changes in disease*

The reader will by now have gained some impression of the amount of work that has already been done. Many paths remain untrodden in both the fields of diagnosis and prognosis. In particular, the visually evoked potential is likely to be a useful index of macular function especially in the light of recent more accurate descriptions of macular disease.

3. *The development of equipment*

In some ways this is the most important and fruitful line of research at present, because the future of electrodiagnosis is going to depend upon the scope for miniaturisation and the use of portable equipment. As hospitals become larger and investigative procedures multiply the need for simple and rapid tests will increase.

If one attempts to project the advances made over the past thirty years into the future, then one can hope for the development of fully portable and hand-held equipment which can be kept in the ophthalmologist's desk. One can hope that remote-controlled sensors will allow us to investigate the function of the retina in the ambulant patient. These advances will not take place without the interest and participation of the clinical ophthalmologist.

Index